# Coping with War-Induced Stress

## The Gulf War and the Israeli Response

# The Plenum Series on Stress and Coping

---

---

# Coping with War-Induced Stress

## The Gulf War and the Israeli Response

### Zahava Solomon

*Tel Aviv University*
*Tel Aviv, Israel*

PLENUM PRESS • NEW YORK AND LONDON

Library of Congress Cataloging-in-Publication Data

On file

ISBN 0-306-44788-6


©1995 Plenum Press, New York
A Division of Plenum Publishing Corporation
233 Spring Street, New York, N.Y. 10013

10 9 8 7 6 5 4 3 2 1

Printed in the United States of America

To my children, Shiry and Ory

May you, and all the children of the world,
never again know war

# Foreword

In the wake of an earlier book (Solomon, 1993), this new work, *Coping with War-Induced Stress: The Gulf War and the Israeli Response,* promises to make Zahava Solomon a modern maven with respect to the psychological effects of war. Dr. Solomon is a high-ranking officer, serving as a psychiatric epidemiologist in the Mental Health Department of the Israeli Defense Forces Medical Corps. She also teaches at Tel Aviv University.

The earlier book dealt with the reactions of the Israeli Defense Forces to the 1982 war in Lebanon, which divided the population of Israel concerning its wisdom and justification. The new book deals with the emotional consequences of the United Nations effort against Iraq after its invasion of Kuwait. Because Israel agreed not to participate actively so as not to endanger the fragile Arab coalition against Iraq, it was in a sense a nonwar—as Solomon refers to it—yet with many features of a war. Although they had quite limited casualties, largely in the Tel Aviv area, the Israelis faced the actuality of damaging Scud missile attacks and the threat that these missiles could not only be targeted to much of Israel but also carry poison gas to other Israeli cities.

Solomon has written a fascinating book about this crisis in Israeli life. In the intimate style of her first book, it is an unusual combination of a remarkable amount of research done by Israeli psychologists and psychiatrists—which Solomon has brought together here—and an absorbing narrative of what was going on before and during the Scud missile attacks and how people dealt with these events. The intimacy comes from the fact that the author was not only a professional psychologist with the defense forces but also an individual with a military husband, herself living the events she writes about. The narrative is written gracefully and engagingly.

The portrait of what happened comes, in effect, from a participant observer who draws together the psychological issues and research done during the Gulf War, as it came to be called. Under continuing stress, much of the research—as Solomon acknowledges—comes from hasty surveys and efforts by psychologists to examine events as they happened, and so much of it lacks the precision and completeness of research designs a scientist would usually prefer. Most such research, however, takes place after the events happen, so the scientific gain could be every bit as great as the loss. The limitations of the research notwithstanding, Solomon has done a remarkable job of making sense of whatever data were available and providing alternative interpretations where they might be indicated.

The 10 chapters of the book center largely on the psychological reactions of different subpopulations in Israel. In addition to surveys applying to the general population, the chapters deal with gender differences, effects on families huddling together in sealed rooms and struggling with gas masks (in the stress of the moment, some people died of asphyxiation because they failed to remove a protective cover), the cramped space and forced intimacy of these rooms, the vulnerable children, senior citizens including Holocaust survivors, those who were casualties of the bombings, the mentally ill, and men who, as soldiers, normally active in combat operations during wartime, were forced by the international agreement to remain passive in the Gulf War.

Although all the topics addressed are important, certain lessons of Solomon's account impress me as especially noteworthy. First, since destruction and casualties were very light, this was a war experience that—except for the direct casualties—was almost entirely psychological. Collectively, its primary quality was not so much one of tragedy and loss but of the threat of loss and the anxiety associated with this threat. In addition, there was the need to cope with diverse sources of physical and psychological stress in an inherently ambiguous situation, expressed both in protective action and in the management of the emotional distress that flows from major stresses.

Second, the experience changed over time. There was an uneasy prelude in which the American and UN reaction to Iraq's invasion of Kuwait remained unclear for 5½ months of uneasy waiting. Then came the Scud missile attacks. There was also some eventual habituation to the bombings, gas masks, and sealed rooms to which families repaired when warnings of an attack came, to the reversals of male and female roles, and to other sources of stress. As Israelis became more experienced with each of the 18 Scud missile attacks, and learned to cope with them and their consequences, their expectations began to change. Habituation really means active coping and changed interpretations of what has happened and what is going to happen. Researchers could and did examine some of the ways people coped with these and other threats; to Solomon's credit and that of the Israeli researchers, the book focuses considerable attention on the coping process, studied usually by means of interview, survey, and observation.

Third, I am struck by the way Solomon deals with what she calls the "myth of panic"—that is, the expectation that panic would occur in large segments of the society under conditions of relative helplessness to life-threatening conditions. Although there was much existential anxiety—about the danger to life and limb, homes, institutions, and threats to society itself—and there were symptomatic, somatic, and emotional evidences of strain, there was no general panic, no social disintegration. People kept their heads, and did what they could to cope. This rule even applied, in the main, to those who suffered from mental illness, and even to most of the children—a group one would expect to be highly vulnerable—who failed to show severe symptoms of stress in the short run, and especially in the long run.

Fourth, since much of the research on the effects of the Gulf War permits comparison of the reactions of different individuals and social groups, it provides an impressive example of individual and group differences in stress reactions and coping patterns. Solomon helps us see that the reactions to stress depended on a wide variety of situational and personality factors. The primary casualties of the Scud attacks—those whose homes were destroyed, who lost loved ones, and who were seriously injured—suffered psychologically more than others at some remove from the dangers and damage.

Finally, the discussion of the role of professional psychologists, psychiatrists, and social workers is a unique contribution to understanding how a society reacts to crisis. I have never before seen an account of professionals speaking to the public in the media, and of reactions to their messages. The media were inundated with professional workers providing information, advice, and opinions about the emotional issues generated by the war. Solomon gives us graphic descriptions of what was said on radio, television, and newspapers by diverse professionals. They also manned hotlines to calm fears and offer suggestions about what to do.

At the same time, and although the public reaction was generally favorable, there was a barrage of criticism about the messages that were relayed in these public presentations because these messages touched on social and political values. Some complained that, although the messages might have helped certain vulnerable people, the welter of reassurances accentuated rather than calmed the anxieties of the population. Others complained that instead of suggesting that anxiety was normal and appropriate—and even that not to be anxious was crazy—people should have been enjoined by the professionals and the government to remain strong and resolute against the threats.

As I read the accounts Solomon provides of the professional messages, and the criticisms and defenses of them, I became aware for the first time of the rich set of controversial issues inherent in crisis situations in which professionals are allowed—in accordance with their individual outlooks—to speak to the public about a shared emotional crisis. Few observers anywhere have given thought to the content of public pronouncements about a common danger. To whom should they be directed? What should be the guiding metatheory? How much should the government—which in Israel did not participate—do to add its own moral or political voice in such situations, not only in Israel, but also in any society facing crisis? These are issues for professionals everywhere to ponder, and the story told by Solomon about what happened is fascinating.

I want also to comment on the great volume of research Israeli psychologists performed during the brief period of the Gulf War. In 1974, shortly after the Yom Kippur War (which greatly troubled Israelis, because prior to this experience they had thought their military might made them invincible), I was one of a number of psychologists who participated in an international research conference in Tel Aviv with the awkward but descriptive title, "Psychological Stress and Adjustment in Time of War and Peace." Two other such conferences followed.

In the address I gave at this conference, which was later published (Lazarus, 1986), I stated that, beset constantly by wars resulting from hostile Arab countries surrounding Israel, this country was a "natural laboratory" for research on stress and coping. Solomon picks up on this theme in her book.

As an American living in relative safety, I had worried about making this statement. Perhaps to people directly facing the problems of frequent warfare and the loss of loved ones, the suggestion that Israeli psychologists were in a remarkable position to study practical issues of stress and coping would seem too clinical and detached.

However, happily for my standing in Israel, Israelis seem to have taken what I said in the realistic and supportive spirit in which it was offered. Indeed, from the large volume of continuing research in Israel on stress and coping—much of it war-related—my statement and the three conferences about stress and coping issues (which began in the mid-1970s) were prescient about the research that would follow. After all, in a country besieged by hostile forces all around it, with a population so small that any losses of its people are deeply felt, defending itself against the ravages of war ought to be highly salient. In any case, Israeli psychologists continue to lead the world in the extent of their research on the psychological consequences and coping processes of war and its aftermath.

This dominant interest certainly applies also to Zahava Solomon and her two recent books. I am confident that those interested in stress and coping will want to read *Coping with War-Induced Stress: The Gulf War and the Israeli Response* as an important societal case history, and as an absorbing and thoughtful account of individual and familial experiences in war and of the stresses it generates.

## REFERENCES

Lazarus, R. S. (1986). The psychology of stress and coping. In C. D. Spielberger & I. G. Sarason (Eds.), *Stress and anxiety, Vol. 10; A sourcebook of theory and research* (pp. 399–418). Washington, D.C.: Hemisphere.
Solomon, Z. (1993). *Combat stress reaction: The enduring toll of war.* New York: Plenum.

RICHARD S. LAZARUS
*University of California*
*Berkeley, California*

# Preface

The Gulf War was the sixth war I experienced in my 41 years. During the 1967 Six Day War, I was a 17-year-old high school student. The Yom Kippur War in 1973 found me a young bride with a husband on the front. By the Lebanon War in 1982, I was the mother of two young children and an officer in the Israel Defense Forces. The Gulf War caught me in midlife: I had been married for 19 years, was the mother of two adolescents, and was caring for my own aging, widowed mother. I was now head of research in the Medical Corps Department of Mental Health.

The months between August 1990, when the Iraqis invaded Kuwait, and the outbreak of the war in January 1991 were full of tension and uncertainty. In August, as instructed by the authorities, my children and I started to prepare for war by buying bicarbonate of soda. Aside from that, our lives proceeded as usual. Though we were apprehensive, we coped through denial. We told ourselves, "Nothing will happen." When we were called to have our gas masks fitted, the children and I had to pressure my husband before he agreed to go. I myself remained surprisingly calm, though as the clock ticked on the American ultimatum, the newspapers published increasingly horrific scenarios of what could happen in the event of a chemical attack and many people were gripped by anxiety.

Then, at 2 a.m. on January 16, our telephone rang. I was informed that the war had started and was summoned to the base. I left my husband and children in bed, put on my uniform, and drove to the base in Tel-Hashomer, passing through the red lights—as did the other cars on the road. At the base I joined the other officers who had been called.

Once there, though, we did not know what to do. Waiting for something to happen, waiting for orders, we stood about in the office of the head of the department, watching the news on the television set that had been brought in for the occasion. The following days were divided between the army base and my base at home. While I was at work, I worried about my children, who were home with their father, and even more about my mother, who had moved in with us. At night I drove home without a gas mask, feeling totally unprotected, since army regulations required that the masks be left at the base.

When the air-raid sirens sounded, we dashed for our "sealed" room. It was only after the war broke out that my husband agreed to comply with the instructions to seal a room by taping plastic sheeting over the windows. We chose our daughter's 3 m × 3 m room, and brought in a television set, a box with food, and bottled water, the regulation pail and wet rag to stuff up the crack at the bottom of the door, and our son's hamster. A radio was already part of the furnishings. Crowded in, we were 11 in number: my husband, children, mother, and I were joined by a neighbor and her two daughters as well as by my sister, her husband, and their four-year-old son.

My husband, Reuven, was our rock, our security. It was he who calmly and methodically sealed the door as our neighbor's nine-year-old daughter agitated; he who removed the protective cap from my mother's gas mask as she huddled in the corner; and he who helped everyone else fit their masks before putting on his own. At first, his unperturbed deliberation was infuriating. Soon it became the stabilizing force in the room. But, in fact, everyone did his or her part. The older kids looked after the younger ones. We played cards and counted the "booms" after the missiles landed. It all soon became routine.

As for myself, I had come a long way since the Six Day War in 1967, when I was a terrified adolescent. I practiced what I had been teaching my students at Tel Aviv University about coping with stressful situations. I was responsible for others, busy organizing our suddenly expanded household, seeing to it that there was food, and doing the washing and cleaning. The responsibility and the activity helped me keep calm.

Also, spending so much time with my mother and sister, with whom I had not lived for 19 years, was wonderful despite the crowding and extra work. There was a sense of sharing and closeness. In the mornings my mother stayed with the three grandchildren while my sister and her husband, and Reuven and I, went to work. In the evenings, we all stayed home together and did not go out or have guests. After each missile attack, I served a snack to make us feel better. At the beginning of February, we even threw a birthday party for my sister. Things were going so well that Reuven took off for Europe for a week-long business trip as if nothing out of the ordinary were happening.

In the army, there was little to do, though we all spent long hours there. We were too preoccupied with the war to go on with our ordinary tasks. New orders were not forthcoming. The daily staff meetings did not alleviate the tension or tedium, and I thought they were pointless.

The one positive thing I can say about the experience is that in the long hours of idleness, I called to mind the work of Philip Saigh, who researched the reactions of the civilian population in Lebanon during the 1982 Israel–Lebanon War. In a way, Saigh was my counterpart; he studied the Lebanese psychiatric victims of the war about whose Israeli victims I had just completed a book. Without having met him, I felt close to him. What I most admired about Saigh's studies was that they were carried out in real time.

While waiting at the base, worrying about my mother and kids and generally being at loose ends, it was hard for me to avoid the thought that the Gulf War—like the Lebanon War 10 years earlier—offered me an opportunity to study the psychological reactions of people to real-life stress under real-time conditions. But something was stopping me. It seemed cynical to take advantage of the situation to further my career. Most research on the psychological effects of national disasters are carried out post hoc. Catastrophic events are usually short-lived and unpredictable and, while they last, everyone is busy surviving. Mental health professionals in an area hit by a disaster are supposed to spend their time minimizing the pathogenic effects of the stressor, not researching it. My feelings were that there was something immoral in "benefiting" from the situation we were in.

Fortunately, early in the war, Yuval Neria, a colleague and a friend, persuaded me otherwise. The war was forced on us, he argued. There was nothing that I or anyone else could do about it. I might as well get something useful out of it for myself and for all those who might benefit from a better understanding of how war affects a civilian population. The research I carried out during the rest of the war was my way of coping with the uncertainties of these days. It helped me get through this period with relative equanimity.

The war ended anticlimactically, and within a few days it seemed as if it had never occurred. It was as if the entire country forgot or suppressed the experience. There were no celebrations, as after the Six Day War; no soul searching, as after the Yom Kippur War; and no political debates, as after the Lebanon War. It was as if the entire six weeks the war lasted had evaporated into thin air.

Mental health professionals were no different. Many of us who had conducted research during the war put our findings in our desk drawers without writing them up or publishing them. There were few conferences on the war, and those that were held attracted few participants. It was only about a half-year after the war ended, on the eve of Rosh Hashanah (the Jewish new year), which is a time of soul searching, that I finally felt ready to confront the war and to write this book.

Chapter 1 provides a descriptive account of the Israeli experience of the war. It describes the mounting tension in Israel during the long waiting period between Iraq's invasion of Kuwait and the expiration of the American ultimatum, focusing on the terrible uncertainty and fear in face of the threat of chemical and gas attack. It then goes on to describe how Israelis lived during the six-week war, during which the population was subjected to 18 separate missile attacks. It describes the "emergency routine" that had everyone at home under voluntary curfew by sundown, when the Scuds began to fall, and the race to the supposedly gas-proofed "sealed room" when the air-raid alarms sounded. It tells of the dilemma of whether to seek protection in the "sealed room" or to go to traditional bomb shelters when it turned out that the Scuds bore conventional warheads, and it relates the feeling of being "sitting ducks" because of the government's policy of restraint.

Chapter 2 presents the results of numerous studies of Israelis' morale, anxiety level, coping patterns, sleep patterns, hospital admissions, mortality, and other indicators of stress during the period in question. Findings showed both heightened distress, with occasional instances of persons literally dying of fright, and a trend of habituation, where people became less and less anxious as the war proceeded.

Chapter 3 presents descriptions and research findings of the various ways in which Israeli families coped with both missile attacks and the "forced intimacy" imposed on them by the nightly curfew. Chapter 4 focuses on gender differences during the war. It shows how men and women had to deal with different stressors, even though they were both part of the same civilian population, and describes the differences in their coping and responses. Chapter 5 presents a large range of empirical studies of Israeli children, from newborns through late adolescents, during and after the war. On the whole, the findings showed that children, like their parents, became habituated to the threat.

Each of the next four chapters deals with a specific high-risk group. Chapter 6 concentrates on aging Holocaust survivors, for whom the Gulf War, with its threat of gas attacks, evoked strong associations with the Nazi years. Survivors' testimonies, clinical impressions, and an empirical study comparing survivors' responses to those of other elderly Israelis suggest that their prior trauma rendered the survivors more vulnerable.

Chapter 7 presents the plight of the "evacuees," whose homes were destroyed in missile attacks and who had to be relocated. It shows that some of those who lost their homes sustained posttraumatic reactions, but that both short- and long-term reactions also depended on the victims' socioeconomic status and the quality of the treatment and accommodations they received. Chapter 8 looks at the mentally ill in Israel's psychiatric hospitals. Both empirical findings and clinical observations indicated that, with the exception of a very small number of persons in whom the war may have triggered or unmasked psychosis, there was no noticeable impairment in the status of any of the chronic patients, and acute schizophrenics became more reality oriented. Chapter 9 deals with Israel's soldiers, who were in the frustrating position of looking on idly while Iraqis launched their attacks. A variety of studies show that although they coped with the forced passivity, they were worried about their families, and that some soldiers suffered reactivation of stress responses from earlier wars.

Chapter 10, the final chapter, examines the role of Israel's mental health professionals during the war. In an effort to contribute, many professionals went public, giving out advice on how to cope with the tensions of the war—on telephone hotlines, in newspaper articles, and on radio and television programs. The chapter describes these activities and discusses the controversy surrounding them, as well as the question of the role that mental health professionals should play in large-scale, public disasters.

# Acknowledgments

This book is based on the research findings and clinical impressions of dozens of mental health professionals in Israel. Data were collected during and after the Gulf War. Some of the studies were carried out by my colleagues and me; others were put at my disposal by the researchers.

With my friend Ed Prager of the Bob Shapell School of Social Work at Tel Aviv University, I collaborated in studying the psychological reactions of elderly Holocaust survivors. My long-time colleagues, Joseph Schwarzwald and Matisyohu Weisenberg of the Psychology Department at Bar Ilan University, worked with me investigating children's coping during the war. Nati Laor, who heads the Ramat Chen Psychiatric Clinic, and Ora Hadar and David Weiler of the Social Services of Ramat Gan, helped me gain access to the wartime evacuees we studied. Avi Bleich, Haim Margalit, Ze'ev Kaplan, and Yafa Singer, my colleagues at the Israel Defense Forces' Mental Health Department, were instrumental in the studies of Israeli soldiers who were consigned to passivity as Iraqi missiles struck the country. With Avner Elizur and Yuval Melamed, I investigated the coping of psychiatric patients during and after the war.

All of these studies carried out during the war were made possible with the support and generous assistance of the Israeli Ministry of Health and the U.S. National Institute of Mental Health. All thanks go to Oded Abramski, former chief scientist of the Ministry of Health, and Susan Solomon, chief of Violence and Traumatic Stress Research Branch at the U.S. National Institute of Mental Health, who helped fund our applications.

I also wish to thank the many individuals in Israel's universities, hospitals, and research institutes, as well as in the Israel Defense Forces, who permitted me to use their research in this book. To my surprise, many of their studies were never written up for publication. Yet not one person I turned to refused to let me see and cite his or her work. I am grateful to every one of these researchers and clinicians for their largesse in contributing to this book.

Finally, I wish to thank Karni Ginzburg, Shira Hantman, and Mark Waysman for helping me collect and organize the material. And I extend special appreciation to Toby Mostysser for her thorough work and penetrating insights in rewriting and editing the manuscript.

# Contents

# 1

# The War That Was Not a War

In retrospect, *the Gulf War*, so termed by Israel, was a misnomer. Israel was not engaged in fighting and, as far as war goes, suffered comparatively little damage. In the 42 days of *Desert Storm*—the American appellation—39 missiles were fired at Israel in 18 separate attacks. But only two people died in direct hits, with another seven asphyxiated in their gas masks. Of the 1,035 injuries that were recorded, the vast majority were minor cuts and bruises. Property damage was also fairly contained. Most of the destruction was concentrated in a number of discrete areas. The hundreds of people who saw their homes demolished, in whole or in part, undoubtedly suffered serious distress. But none of them was left out in the winter cold; all were accommodated in hotels at government expense until their homes were refurbished or alternative ones found. Israel's infrastructure remained intact, and its public hospitals and war-related social services continued to function. While the bombed-out inhabitants of Baghdad huddled without electricity and water and endured shortages from food to fuel, Israelis wanted for little and, as time passed, increasingly resumed their former activities.

Yet, this "war" or "storm," however one wishes to describe it, was so stressful, so terrifying, that six months after the demon Saddam Hussein was safely put back into his bottle, Israelis who had locked away their fear and gone back to work and school or were planning their summer vacations began saying to one another, "What did you do during the war?" "Do you remember . . .?" "I was so scared that . . ." and are still swapping stories as this book is being written two years later. If any experience characterized this war–nonwar for Israelis, it was fear, a

1

pervasive, inveigling fear, all the more disturbing, embarrassing even, because it had so little concreteness in which to wrap itself.

What made this war that was not a war so frightening? What was it that so disoriented, so threw off balance, a nation as battle-practiced as Israel—whose soldiers bravely fight an average of two wars per generation and whose citizens have learned to adjust to the constant threat and reality of terrorist attacks?

The answer, or answers, to this question may be found in two places. One is in the peculiar nature of the war itself, over which Israel had very little control. The other is in the policy of denial that Israel's leaders adopted, which wrought confusion and exacerbated people's apprehensions both in the course of the war and in the five-and-a-half-month prelude that led up to it.

## THE LONG PRELUDE

In Israel, Saddam Hussein's attack on Kuwait on August 2, 1990, ushered in a period that can be likened to a long, tense plucking of daisy petals, only with the vital concern not the romantic "he loves me, he loves me not" but two interrelated "will he or will he not?" questions bearing not on love but on life: Will the Iraqi dictator Saddam Hussein withdraw from Kuwait? Will U.S. president George Bush stand by his ultimatum to make him? A host of questions associated with these two questions arose, all culminating in the question: What will be the implications for Israel?

From the first, Saddam tried to implicate Israel in the imbroglio. He started immediately after the annexation of Kuwait with accusations that the combat planes the United States had sent to the Gulf were Israeli planes painted over with U.S. insignia. Posing as the liberator of the Palestinians, he tried to "link" any withdrawal from Kuwait to Israel's withdrawing from the administered territories. He moved missiles toward Israel, and he made repeated threats to strike at Israel's civilian population. Yet, until the 2 A.M. air strike against Iraq by the American-led coalition on the morning of January 16, no one was absolutely sure that there would be war. And not until Iraq's Scud missile attack on the Tel Aviv and Haifa areas two nights later was it certain that he would—or could—make good on his threat to attack Israel.

For five and a half months, Israelis were poised on a kind of emotional see-saw. With every international effort to pry Saddam out of Kuwait, it seemed that war might be averted. The Security Council embargo might work. The Arabs themselves might succeed in coaxing him out. Evidence that Bush was succeeding in gathering a coalition might persuade Saddam to withdraw his troops. The Bush-orchestrated United Nations' ultimatum might do it. Then, as it became plain that Saddam was not to be dissuaded by military threat and that Western hopes were pinned on various diplomatic efforts, Israelis rightly or wrongly began to sniff appeasement. There was fear that the war-wary West would buy Saddam's linkage or that U.S. Secretary of State James Baker might make concessions at Israel's expense. And when he did not, but France and Germany made last-minute efforts to avert a confrontation, the fear was that they would be the ones to sell Israel down the river.

As the ultimatum date approached, many Israelis didn't know which would be worse: an immediate war, in which the use of unconventional weapons could lead to anything from large-scale injuries to the Israeli population to worldwide ecological disaster, or some temporary settlement that would pry Saddam out of Kuwait but leave him in office to build up his destructive capacities. To the fear of war was added the fear that there might not be a war: that Bush and the European Allies would buckle under mounting antiwar pressure in their home countries and arrive at some face-saving compromise at Israel's expense or, that if they did attack, they might limit their campaign to the Iraqi troops in Kuwait, leaving the dictator intact with all his military might. To the question of whether there would be war was added the dilemma of which would be worse: a war fought now by the American-led coalition but with unknown consequences for Israel or a war a few years later against a stronger, nuclear-equipped tyrant, which Israel might be left to fight on its own.

Throughout these five and a half months, every international effort and every wily response by Saddam provoked new anxieties. At the core of them all was the one great threat that differentiated this war from every anxiety-provoking war Israel had fought in the past: the threat of chemical and biological attack against the civilian population. Saddam introduced the threat early in August in general terms when he warned that he would meet any U.S. action against Iraq with a strike against Israel. Later in the month, his foreign minister Tariq Aziz proclaimed that Iraq would use chemical weapons should Israel resort to nuclear ones, which Israel had never threatened to do. The Iraqi threats were repeated at various intervals and escalated with the proclamation that Saddam would incinerate half of Israel and had the weapons to do it. Though unsubstantiated, the boasts could not be discounted. The Iraqi dictator had proved his capacity to use gas in the war against Iran and, when that was over, against the unprotected Kurds in his own country.

The television and newspaper pictures of gassed Iranian soldiers and stricken Kurdish villagers left little doubt about his readiness and ability to use such weapons. All in all, he mounted a remarkably effective fear campaign. Western intelligence overestimated his troop strength and military capacity. Israelis were taken in by his demonic self-aggrandizement, as were many Americans and Europeans who were not in the line of fire.

The threat of chemical and biological attack was terrifying. Unlike conventional weapons, the damage that these amorphous agents of destruction could inflict was little known and seemed to be potentially boundless. The pictures of Saddam's gas victims told of its immediate power. Even more frightening was the specter of unknown, long-term injury: of lifelong infirmity or slow death through disease and chemical poisoning; of contaminated air, water, land, and food; of genetic deformities passed from generation to generation. The ordinary person, even the generally well educated, had little idea of the nature and scope of the power of these weapons: exactly what the weapons could do to them, what distances their effect might spread, how long their poison might linger on in the environment. Where facts were sparse, imagination filled in with a vengeance.

Adding to the anxiety was the fear that there was little protection against the invidious penetration of chemicals and germs. In previous wars, Israel's highly effective antiaircraft defenses kept most enemy planes from crossing the country's borders and gave the civilian population a sense of being shielded. These defenses would be of little use against missiles, however, and everyone knew it. Nor, Israelis were told, would their air-raid shelters provide much protection against missile-propelled gas. Designed for conventional airplane bombings, they were ground-floor shelters, located in apartment buildings, in newer office buildings, or in older neighborhoods. For conventional bombings, there was enough warning time to reach these shelters, and their reinforced concrete walls provided protection against blasts. The possibility of missile-delivered chemical payloads made these shelters dangerous, however. With the short warning time, there was the danger that people would be struck en route (as actually happened). And since the destructive agents in the gas were likely to sink, it was safer to be on higher ground.

At the same time, Israel was deprived of its major traditional defense: the power to take military action. This defense had served it well in the 1967 Six Day War, when Israel knocked out the entire Egyptian air force before it even got off the ground. More recently, it had served well when, under Menachem Begin, an Israeli air strike knocked out Iraq's nuclear reactor. But now, early on in the Gulf crisis, Israel was consigned to a watch-and-wait position. The coalition set up by President Bush was predicated on Israel's total exclusion, not only from the coalition itself but also from any military action. Israel was warned to keep a low profile lest it taint the anti-Saddam campaign with Zionist motives and lead to the defection of the Arab members, who for the first time in modern history were joined with the Western world against one of their own. This meant that there could be no large preemptive attack, no small-scale operation against Iraq's chemical arsenals, and, worse, no military response should the Iraqi dictator strike.

Israel's citizens and government understood the logic of this approach, and it is doubtful that many hankered for yet another war. Also, to sweeten the pill, the Americans promised to come to Israel's aid should it be attacked by Iraq and to keep a U. S. troop presence after the crisis was resolved. So the public went along, and Israel's leaders took care to stress that Israel was not a party to the fray. Yet the policy meant that unless things got very bad indeed, Israel could not take action to defend itself. To make doubly sure of this, the Americans steadfastly refused Israel real-time satellite information on Iraqi missile movements. Israel's hands were tied and, for the first time in its modern history, the safety of its citizens was entrusted to the good will and ability of others, of which most Israelis are most skeptical.

The anxieties generated by the threat of unconventional weapons and the constraints on self-defense were not the whole picture, however. At every level, from the military through the general public, there were contradictory assessments. While some predicted doom, others averred that nothing of consequence would happen, that there would be no war, and that if there were, Saddam, for all his threats, would not be able to hit Israel. Two notable examples of the latter can be recalled from the week of January 15, just before the ultimatum ran out. One was the television appearance of a respected historian, who, the day before war broke out, declared in a tone of certainty that he will never live down, that not a single Iraqi missile would penetrate Israeli air space. The other was a sardonic remark, also on a television talk show, by the generally laconic former chief of staff Rafael Eitan. By that time, Israelis were making preparations for attack (of which more will be said shortly), cross-taping the windows of their homes in case of conventional attack and preparing "sealed rooms" in case of gas and chemicals. With equal certainty, Eitan dismissed the activity as "therapy" for people whose anxiety was supposedly "neurotic."

Given this complex of circumstances—the uncertainty of war, the fearful unknowns of chemical weaponry, the enforced military passivity, and questions about Iraq's power—Israel's options were limited to making preparation for contingencies, to if–then scenarios where both propositions were difficult to delineate and articulate. More than in ordinary times, it was left for Israel's strife-ridden government to provide definition: to say this is the situation, these are the possibilities, this is what is being done. Instead, major government figures kept a low profile. There were repeated and expected threats that Israel would know how to respond should Iraq be so foolish as to cross some red line, presumably the use of gas or biological weaponry. But there was no calling together of the nation, no Churchillian voice. The vacuum was filled by academicians, journalists, and other media-made "experts" who aired a wide variety of predictions on radio and television, fanning the speculation and adding to the tension.

The decision to prepare the population for chemical attack was made against the background of the uncertainties described above. In the course of the waiting period, preparations were made on several fronts: detoxification and triage and treatment plans were drawn up for all hospitals and medical centers in Israel; instructions were issued for preparing a "sealed room" in people's homes; and protective kits were supplied to the entire civilian population, containing gas masks tailored to the various needs of babies, young children, the elderly, men with beards, and people with allergies and pulmonary diseases, and syringes of the detoxicant atropine with doses calibrated to different age groups. Along with this there was a nationwide educational effort aimed at teaching the proper use of the gas kits and avoiding accidents. Nonetheless, it is precisely in the matter of these protective measures where the confusion that beset the leadership was expressed.

Distribution of the gas kits was delayed by a lengthy debate, not only about their necessity but also about the timing. On the one side were arguments for distributing the masks early on in the crisis along with detailed information about them and training in their use. The view here was that the better prepared the population, the less damage there would be in the event of chemical warfare. Well-informed, well-practiced people would be better able to use the protective kits properly and better know how to respond to the different situations that might arise. They would also feel more secure. There was also the point that it was better to distribute the protective kits at leisure and when people were still relatively calm than in a last-minute rush, when people were afraid of imminent attack. On the other hand were arguments for delaying the distribution of protective kits until close to the time when they might be needed. These included the argument that early distribution would bring home the chemical threat, provoking panic and undermining tourism and the rest of Israel's wobbly economy. It was also argued that if the kits were put in the hands of the civilian population, they would be mishandled and unfit for use when needed.

The debate, like the one about whether Israel would be attacked and, if so, by what kind of weapons, ran through every level of the government and the military, including the mental health agencies. In the end, a compromise route was followed. In October, the government finally decided to distribute the kits, for the first time acknowledging the possibility that the threat was real. Distribution centers were set up in schools, community centers, and other public places, and young conscripts were swiftly trained to teach the use of the masks. However, the training was shallow and merely theoretical. Instruction was carried out in groups, with as many as 40 or more participants, who were shown how to put on the masks and told when and how to inject themselves with the atropine that was provided in a neatly packaged syringe. Invariably, a bemused or bewildered audience respectfully strained to follow as their young instructors removed caps, adjusted straps, and fit the somewhat complicated apparatus on the head of an obliging volunteer. They were warned not to open their own kits until further instructions. Nor were sample masks provided for them to try on or even touch. The demonstrations took all of 15 to 20 minutes. The outcome was that many people were caught in a quandary when they had to put their gas masks on for the first time in the wee hours of the night. The deaths by gas mask asphyxiation could be attributed to the poor training. Fortunately, there was one exception to this policy. The schools provided hands-on training that enabled their students to drill donning their masks and following the various emergency instructions. This proved itself during the first strike when, in more than a few families, the children assisted their parents instead of the other way around (Noy, 1991).

For most of the period preceding the Coalition invasion, things were kept on what Israelis call "a low burner," a bit like the Sabbath *cholent* (Jewish peasant stew, customarily prepared for Sabbath meals). Certain segments of the military, especially the air force, were calling up reserves and visibly making preparations. But, in general, the spirit of denial filtered down from the upper echelons to the general public, who went about its business apparently unperturbed until very close to the January 15 deadline. The fear that surfaced then was subdued. There was little stocking up, and some people didn't even bother to get their gas masks when they were first distributed.

The result was a last-minute dash and frenzy. As the date approached, military and civil defense authorities moved into action. The public were instructed to prepare a "sealed room" in which they could secure themselves in case of chemical attack. The room was to be stocked with bottled water and canned and other hermetically sealed foodstuffs, and gas-proofed by taping plastic sheeting over the windows and air-conditioning vents. The effectiveness of these rooms was never tested in this war, but to many, especially to those with battle experience and familiar with the force of aerial bombardment, the procedure smacked of the ridiculous.

Suddenly, too, television, radio, and newspaper space was given over to civil defense instructions: how to use the gas kits, how to make and equip the sealed room, what to do when the air-raid sirens sounded. People who had not bothered preparing in advance made a beeline for the hardware stores and supermarkets. Masking tape and nylon sheeting that had been lying around for months shot up in price until they disappeared from the shelves, and factories went into night shifts to make more. Baking soda, which was recommended as a remedy for chemical poisoning, couldn't be bought at any price. Bottled water was in short supply.

There was also a lot of last-minute confusion related to the gas masks. For example, the authorities decided to switch the gas masks designated for young children from a "passive" to a battery-driven "active" type, which pumped filtered air into the sealed hood. Parents were advised to pick up replacements, but the new masks were available only for certain areas. This created unease both in the parents whose children kept the old mask (If it's any good, why are they changing the others?) and in those whose children were to be issued the improved models (What other mistakes aren't they telling us about?). The week before January 15, the latter joined crowds of others, from people with allergy and heart problems, who also required "active" masks, to the simply negligent, who had not picked up their kits when they were first distributed, in long, pushing lines, waiting several hours in a few reopened distribution centers.

In the last days before the ultimatum ran out, the tension culminated in scenes at the airport, where first tourists and other foreigners and then Israelis crowded for a flight out. On January 14, about 14,000 people left the country. The flight of Israelis before a war was a truly extraordinary event. In every previous war, Israelis had stayed put, and those who were abroad came rushing back. They stayed or flocked back before the 1967 war, when people were afraid that the country would be overrun, and some even expected another holocaust. They stayed or returned during the 1973 war, when the Egyptians had succeeded in crossing the Suez Canal and the Syrians in taking back part of the Golan that had been wrested from them in 1967. Being in Israel during wartime had been a matter of widely accepted principle for soldiers and

civilians alike, which expressed commitment to the country and identification with one of its basic tenets: that Israel is the rightful and only
secure home of the Jewish people. In earlier wars, there were even
Diaspora Jews who came to Israel for the express purpose of taking part
in the war effort.

The departures, which were aired on radio and television, had an
embarrassed, even shameful, quality. Relatively few of those who were
interviewed at the airport admitted outright that they were leaving because they were afraid. Most gave excuses, such as the following: I was
invited to a wedding (bar mitzvah, golden anniversary, and so on)
abroad; the trip was preplanned; my parents (children, friends) who are
living abroad insist that I join them. The excuses were unconvincing.
And as most Israelis were preparing their sealed rooms and cross-taping
their windows with masking tape (in case of conventional attack), those
who were slinking out made those who held their ground—whether out
of identification with the country, a better ability to cope with their fear,
less fear, or lack to choice—wonder whether they were doing the right
thing. The degree to which the exodus reflected the country's diminished social cohesiveness, the terror inspired by the threat of unconventional warfare, or the confusion of the preceding months is a matter of
conjecture. But the five and a half months of uncertainty and denial all
seemed to come to a head in the unprecedented flight of Israelis who,
for the first time in the country's history, were neither in a position to
fight nor convinced that they were properly protected.


## SITTING OUT THE FRAY

On January 16, telephones in Israel began to ring at 2 a.m., when
CNN correspondent Peter Arnett announced the Coalition air attack on
Iraq. The news spread quickly phone to phone, and by the time they
switched on the morning news many, maybe even most, Israelis knew
that war had started. A state of emergency was declared; the public were
told to remain at home, unpack their gas masks, and stay tuned to the
radio for further instructions; schools, universities, and public offices
were closed. Israel's three public radio stations were merged into one
and, together with the two government-run television stations, broadcast
whatever information could be gleaned from the foreign networks. The
first euphoric reports that the Coalition planes were pummeling Iraq
raised people's hopes of a speedy victory but also sparked anxiety. Now
that the attack had started, Israel was in the line of fire.

Apprehension became reality at 2 a.m. on January 17. The hourly news broadcast was interrupted by a hissing code, "nahash tzefa" (viper snake), followed almost immediately by air-raid sirens and by the swoosh and glass-shattering boom of the first Iraqi missiles, six landing in Tel-Aviv, Israel's most populous city, and two in Haifa, in the north of the country. The doubters were proved wrong. The Iraqis could aim and hit.

Practically every important detail that could have gone wrong that predawn did. The air-raid sirens were not properly functioning. In some areas they did not go off at all; in others they sounded so softly that many people slept through them. The warning time was extremely short. In some areas of Tel Aviv, the sirens went off at the same time as, or even after, the missiles landed. Nowhere was there more than 90 seconds' notice. The code "nahash tzefa," which was the signal to sound the sirens, might have informed the nighttime radio buffs, only no one knew what it meant. Then, once people were awake and presumably in their sealed rooms with their gas masks over their mouths and noses and had switched on the radio to find out what was happening, they were treated to almost an hour of chatter and love songs by two apparently unbriefed disc jockeys before Nachman Shai, the army spokesman, came on at 3 a.m. with the announcement that would be repeated 18 times in the following six weeks: "Due to a missile attack on Israel, a real alert has been sounded. All residents must immediately put on their gas masks and close themselves off in their sealed rooms. After the family has entered the room, the doorway should be sealed with masking tape. The air conditioning must be turned off immediately. You must check to see that your children have put their gas masks on properly. Stay tuned to the radio for further announcements" (Kol Israel, IBS, January 17, 1991). It was—and still is—hard to avoid the thought that had this been a gas attack, as expected, there could have been a lot more damage than the 22 wounded persons and several hundred broken windows that were recorded.

The good news that the missiles bore conventional warheads was less reassuring than that fact would be in the aftermath. For the major cause of anxiety, the threat of gas, remained unabated. That this strike was conventional did not mean that others would be. The same applied to the second, third, and fourth strikes, until the very end of the war. The new questions that knotted up people's stomachs were, Why isn't he using gas? Will he use gas? If so, when? Speculation ran from the possibility that the missiles could not hold chemical warheads to the idea that Saddam was deterred by fear of Israeli retaliation, in which case, the unconsoling thought ran, he might switch to chemicals if he were pushed to the brink and felt he had little left to lose.

The fear of gas, then, remained, though with reduced intensity, until the last days of the war, with constant talk of the Iraqi chemical arsenal on the radio and television. In the prime target areas, the Tel Aviv and Haifa metropolitan regions, where most of the Scuds fell, fear continued to affect people's behavior even after the damage that conventional warheads could inflict became clear. With the exception of a fair number of thrill seekers who did things like go up on their roofs to watch the Scuds fall, and some fatalists and macho men who went about without their gas masks, most people in the high-risk areas continued to observe precautions against chemical attack. The majority carried their gas masks with them and put them on when the sirens sounded.

At the same time, a number of strikes in the Tel Aviv region showed the damage that conventional warheads could inflict. The first two strikes, the one that opened the attack on Israel in the dark hours of Friday morning and the one that followed at 7 a.m. that Saturday, caused limited damage: broken windows and shutters and people lightly cut and bruised by the splinters. The third strike a few days later, however, resulted in the total destruction of eight apartment buildings in the small city of Ramat Gan in the greater Tel Aviv area. Walls were torn through, floors were caved in, and most of the buildings were reduced to rubble. The sight on television of the people who, in a flash, had lost their homes and all their possessions, and who were standing shocked or crying amid the debris, sent tremors through people already frightened and on edge. A similar strike eight days later, in which 12 buildings were destroyed, brought the lesson home.

This combination—the amorphous threat of gas with its unknown damage and the shattering reality of conventional attack—characterized the Gulf War in Israel, and it shaped people's behavior and created constant tension for the 42 days that the war lasted.

Much of the tension was concentrated in the sealed room. To begin with, the enormous speed of the missiles made the procedure in the sealed room a frantic race against time. When the siren sounded, children and sometimes old people as well had to be awakened and rushed into the room. Then, once everyone was inside, the sealing of the room had to be completed. As it was, only the windows were sealed, but the door had to be shut and made airtight too. To speed up the process, people were advised to have half-widths of masking tape already stuck onto the door or adjacent frame, so that all that remained to be done was to shut the door, smooth the remaining half-width of tape over the gap, and stuff up the crevice at the bottom with a cloth that had been soaked in a baking soda solution.

The gas masks had to be properly fitted. This meant removing the various protective caps that would asphyxiate you if you left them on, adjusting difficult-to-ply rubber straps, and fitting the mask properly over the head and face. If you had an "active" mask, you also had to buckle a belt with the motor around your waist. School-age children, especially the older ones, who had the benefit of hands-on practice, sometimes came to the aid of their fumbling parents. Younger children generally could not put on their masks by themselves and needed the assistance of parents or older siblings. In families with small children, the adults in the room could divide the labor, one handling the door, the other seeing to the kids. Where there were lots of little ones or only one parent, the pressure was all the greater. To complicate matters, some children were frightened by the masks or so uncomfortable in them that it was a struggle to make them wear them. Infants and babies posed a special challenge. An ingenious boxlike contraption of transparent plastic on a collapsible metal frame had been devised for his or her protection; the problem was that many were loath to get inside, and frantic parents wound up shoving them in screaming and kicking. Moreover, no one really knew which to do first, to seal the room or to get the masks on. During the first few strikes, when the warning time before the strike was only 90 seconds, the whole thing was an impossible mission. When the air-raid signals were finally connected to the U.S. surveillance satellite and the warning time extended to five minutes, it could be done but was still a race against the clock. Some families were able to solve the problem partially by sealing their bedrooms and having the children sleep there or by sealing the children's room. But not everyone could fall back on these solutions.

After everyone was in the room, the room sealed, and the masks all snugly fitted, the waiting came: first for the boom that told of a strike in an area nearby, then for the radio announcement that the missile had fallen. That was followed by a longer wait, when the general area of the attack was announced, and after that, by another wait while the authorities checked whether the warhead was chemical or conventional. Only when that was completed were people released from the rooms, area by area. The time spent in the sealed room was rarely more than 45 minutes at a stretch, but no one could know in advance how long it would be. On some nights there were several alarms (including false ones), so it was in and out again. During those waits, children had to be kept calm and occupied, and the attention of the adults was usually divided between the radio (or television) broadcasts and the kids. Complications could also arise when husband and wife were at odds or when friction with visiting relatives added personal tensions to the ones inherent in the situation. On the other hand, there could be occasions when one or another family member was not at home when the siren sounded, and those in the sealed room were worried for his or her safety.

These pressures of the sealed room might have been more support-
able had everyone felt well protected once they were masked and sealed
inside. They did not. Some were doubtful from the outset. Others felt
increasingly vulnerable as they saw windows and walls blown away by
conventional warheads or by parts of falling Patriot antimissile batteries.
The information was that chemical warheads would not cause the physical destruction that conventional ones did, so that a chemical attack
would leave buildings intact and their occupants safe in their sealed
rooms. But who could guarantee that chemical and conventional weapons would not be trained on the same site?

The damage of the conventional attacks reawakened the prewar
debate, which had never been fully laid to rest, about whether sealed
rooms or conventional shelters offered better protection. The authorities reiterated their prewar argument that because chemical attack could
be expected to cause more injury and death than conventional attack,
and no one could predict in advance when one would occur, the sealed
rooms would save more lives. But there were loud dissenting voices
claiming just the opposite: that more lives would be saved in the shelters.

With their lives on the line and mistrustful of the authorities, Israelis fell back on their own judgment. As the war progressed, more and
more people made a beeline for their shelters when the siren sounded.
The first to do so were people who lived in private houses, who had their
own personal shelters and sealed them to do double duty. Others soon
followed. In apartment buildings, diligent residents sealed the communal ground-floor shelters and the tenants crowded in, fitting their masks
on the way. Those who stayed in the sealed rooms of their apartments
did so for a variety of reasons. Some may have accepted the official
reasoning. Others could not reach their shelters in the requisite time.
These included residents of older neighborhoods, where the shelters
were in some neighborhood facility rather than in the apartment buildings; the elderly, the handicapped, and others who could not bound
down many flights of stairs (using the elevator during an attack was
unsafe and *forbidden*) in time to get into the shelter before the door was
shut; and those who lived in the upper stories of high-rises.

In the course of the war, some of those who could not or would not
go to the shelters but felt unsafe in their flimsy sealed rooms found an
ingenious compromise: they went out into the halls of their apartment
buildings. Many of the halls in the newer buildings were inner spaces
surrounded by apartments and had either no windows or small ones that
could be easily sealed. The features seemed to make them good bets in
case of either conventional or chemical attack, promising protection
without the risk of being caught en route to a shelter. Some people
devised yet a further refinement on this approach—huddling in the hall

for five minutes (in case of conventional attack), then bounding for their sealed rooms, in case the attack were chemical. Initially, the authorities warned against the hallway solution, then eventually gave it their OK. With or without an official blessing, however, this search for solutions, the running from sealed room to shelter or hall and sometimes back to sealed room again, all with the gas mask at hand, grew out of and gave expression to the intense uncertainties that marked this war.

When the missiles began falling, a kind of second exodus started. It began as slow stream after the first strikes in the Tel Aviv area, gathered momentum after the buildings in Ramat Gan were totaled, and swelled to a great flood as the tension of living with the strikes and the uncertainty mounted and the contagion of fear spread. One hundred thousand people in all surged out of Tel Aviv and Ramat Gan (Dolev, 1992). They went to friends and relatives in mosahvim and kibbutzim; to guest houses in the north of the country, usually deserted during the winter lull; to hotels in Jerusalem, which, with its large Arab population in the eastern part of the city, was apparently out of the trajectory of the Iraqi missiles; to the occupied territories, which, at least in the beginning, seemed safe for the same reason; and to the south of the country, especially the resort town of Eilat, where hotels that had been hurt by the pinch on foreign tourism suddenly experienced a grim revival of business. Although these places were less inviting targets than Tel Aviv, they could be considered a safe distance away only in a country of Israel's Lilliputian dimensions.

This second exodus occurred despite the fact that no directives were given to evacuate the city, and, like the first, it had a demoralizing effect on many of those who stayed behind. Tel Aviv's mayor, Shlomo Lahat, called them "deserters" (Derfner, 1991, p. 17). Nor did it necessarily bring peace of mind to those who left. Of these, many soon came back—drawn to the psychological comfort of their homes and belongings or driven back into the cauldron by the strain on their pocketbooks or by the wear and tear of living with people with whom they were not intimate or did not want to be with. About half had come back the third week into the war, when the schools, which had been shut, were reopened, though about a third stayed away until the war's end (Dolev, 1992).

## THE EMERGENCY ROUTINE

The great majority who remained in the high-risk Tel Aviv or Haifa areas, or who returned to them, gradually adjusted to what became known as an "emergency routine." During the first four days of the war, instructions were to stay at home, except for people in essential services, such as medical and military personnel. Thus, with those exceptions, most people were confined to their homes. Those days were particularly tense, not only because they were at the beginning and no one knew what to expect, but also because of the unaccustomed strain of being cooped up indoors with too much anxiety to pursue one's normal activities or to do anything that required concentration. Spouses, kids, and parents, got on each other's nerves, so it was a great relief when people were allowed out again on the fifth day. But what they could and could not do was constrained by the situation, and the oxymoronic "emergency routine" itself created additional stresses.

The government created an impossible situation for families by closing the schools but sending the adults back to work. The return to routine was thus only partial. Where both parents worked, some couples took turns babysitting, others argued about it, and in other families the task fell, as such tasks usually do, to the women.

At home, the days were long, tedious, and tension-ridden. Despite the lifting of the "curfew," parents were reluctant either to let their kids go out by themselves, even to visit friends, or to leave them at home on their own, even to go to the supermarket. So the sense of house arrest persisted. The children, who on many occasions had been awakened the night before by one or more alarms, tended to absorb the adults' anxiety and were often tired, bored, and irritable. Much of the time was occupied with television. The day often began with rapt attention to the televised newscasts—Israel's and CNN's—which recounted in great detail the progress of the Coalition in Iraq and the related events in Israel. Afterward, the television was kept on for entertainment or, more aptly, distraction. Unfortunately, the "great escape" offered only boring talk shows and old reruns. Some of the children's shows tried to relate to the situation, for example by showing a puppet in a gas mask and discussing the subject in terms children could understand; but, in general, the television did not provide much entertainment. Some of the people who packed their bags and left Tel Aviv did so as much to alleviate the tedium and tension of the semiconfinement as to flee the Scuds.

Outside in the office and shop, things were also tense. Employees, who footed the bill for the three days of official absence, had their own worries. To get back their full work force, the larger enterprises and organizations set up day-care facilities (which, unfortunately, did not outlast the war). But the smaller businesses could not do this, and some parents took their kids to work with them. Whole branches of the economy came to a virtual standstill. Construction ceased with the absence of

Arab workers. Industrialists had major difficulties meeting production schedules and were unable to ship what they produced abroad. Small businesses, such as shops and restaurants, saw their customers dwindle. So in addition to being concerned about their safety, many people had real worries about their livelihoods. One of the only branches of the economy that did well was the food business, as people stocked up on nonperishables (canned goods, long-life milk, and so on) and on candy and such to assuage their anxiety.

The decision to reopen the school three weeks into the war eased some of these conflicts, but not totally. Kindergartens and special schools for handicapped children were not reopened. In the schools that were reopened, parents were required to take turns being on hand should an alarm sound and should extra help be needed to get hundreds of children into their gas masks and to the shelters in the requisite five minutes. For parents with a number of children, this duty could take up several mornings a week. Nor was the sight of the schools particularly calming. Before they were reopened, the teachers and staff came in to seal the windows in the classrooms and corridors. But if the sealed rooms at home seemed woefully inadequate, those in the schools, with their profusion of windows and doors, seemed all the more so. Many of the shelters were small for the number of pupils they would have to hold and, in any case, would take some time to reach. So parents who might have been pleased to have their children back in a structured framework could not help worrying about how protected they were should something happen, and some of them opted to keep their kids at home.

Then came the twilight hour. With the exception of the one Saturday morning strike at the beginning of the war, the other attacks all came after dark. The emergence of this pattern was one of the things that made it possible for the schools to reopen and for daytime activities to return to a certain prewar level. But it also led to a mad dash for home come evening. At 5 p.m., shops locked their doors, offices closed, and the roads became one long traffic jam as everyone raced to get home before dark. With everyone leaving their work places at about the same time, the traffic jams were worse than the ones to which Israelis had already become accustomed and made getting home before sunset and "Scud time" all that much harder. The ordinary aggravation of sitting in stalled traffic was also greatly intensified by the fear of not making it home on time and getting caught in one's car in an attack. Cars could be sealed but provided little protection from conventional weapons.

Evenings saw the resumption of a kind of voluntary curfew. Most restaurants, cafés, and movie houses were closed. Those that remained open had few customers. Large public gatherings, such as weddings and bar mitzvahs, were moved up to afternoon hours. People cut down on their evening visiting. At home, many tried to get dinner and showers out of the way early so as not to be caught in the bathroom when an alarm sounded. These measures did not always work.

Even with this partial normalization, the threat of the Scuds remained the dominant fact and major determinant of people's activities. It governed how and where people spent their time. It brought them scurrying back to their homes at sundown. It constantly occupied people's thoughts and demanded decisions at every turn. To take a few of many examples, people kept overnight bags packed next to their beds, so that they could take them and run if they had to; they slept in jogging suits, rather than pajamas, so that they would be in street clothes in the shelters or in case their roofs were blasted away; some had their children sleep in shoes. Moreover, although it turned out that the Scuds continued to arrive only at night, there was nothing to guarantee that the Iraqis would not try to strike in daylight. As people went about with their gas masks in their cars or knocking at their sides, no one knew when a siren might sound and they would have to run for shelter. This concern was always there, persistent and oppressive, however much people adapted themselves to it.

## NEW ROLES AND NEW RULES

In addition to coping with the uncertainties of when and with what Saddam would attack and with the numerous practical spinoffs of the threat, Israelis also had to cope psychologically with the new roles and rules that this unsettling war created. Israelis are accustomed to wars beyond their borders. With the single exception of the 1948 War of Independence, none of Israel's wars prior to the Gulf had been fought on Israeli soil. Israel's defense policy has consistently been to move the battle to enemy territory. This has been the strategy in every war, including the 1973 Yom Kippur War, where Egyptian and Syrian forces succeeded in crossing into the Sinai and Golan, under Israeli control. These forces were quickly routed, and the fight was moved into Egypt and Syria proper before the international community called for a ceasefire.

The Gulf War took place on Israeli soil. And that was not all. It was a war in which civilians were specifically targeted, while Israeli soldiers could not prevent the attacks and were not permitted to retaliate. This turning the other cheek was also a significant departure from many years of precedent. No Israeli government had ever permitted attacks against Israelis to go unpunished before. To take the most clear-cut example, ever since terrorist forces have started using Lebanon as a launching base for rockets against Israel's northern towns, the Israel Defense Forces (IDF) have struck back at the bases and training camps. If this did not always work as a deterrent, it did send the message that Israelis would not be attacked with impunity and gave the targets of the attacks the feeling that the Israeli army was behind them.

This was not the feeling in the Gulf War. Although the air force was on full alert and certain army units were preparing for various contingencies, there was little expectation that the IDF would play an active role. The government's decision to exercise restraint in the face of Iraqi provocations received wide public support, moving from 76% soon after the attacks started to a hefty 81% after they had become a fact of life (Levy, S., 1991a). It was evidently understood that Saddam was trying to goad Israel into belligerency to distract attention from his rape of Kuwait, to make himself the hero of the Arab masses, and to break up the coalition against him.

Yet while it was generally accepted that prudence was the better part of valor, the enforced passivity felt unnatural for Israelis accustomed to action, and it reinforced the sense of helplessness created by the missile attacks. Men who in other wars were on the front (or would have been if they had been the right age) were stuck at home, sealing doors, helping their kids on with their masks, or running to shelters dubiously equipped for chemical attack. Women who had learned to expect their men to protect the family and keep danger at a distance had to readjust their expectations. A going joke was that soldiers on duty were sending care packages home rather than the other way around.

More was involved than the shifting of gender expectations and the reversal of home and front. For hundreds of years Jews in the Diaspora had been victimized because they did not carry arms and did not fight. The pogroms of Europe typically had bands of armed bullies pillaging, raping, and murdering unarmed Jews huddled in boarded-up homes that offered little protection, while the men of the family were as powerless to avert the disaster as their women and children. In the Holocaust, which is part and parcel of Israeli consciousness, the violence reached genocidal proportions, with unarmed and dispirited Jews forced to dig their own graves or walk into gas chambers. Israel was conceived of by its founders and early pioneers as a place where such things would not happen, and generations of Israeli schoolchildren were taught as much. It would not happen because in their own state Jews would be able to bear arms and fight back. For over 40 years, the Israeli army, a broad-based citizens' army and one of the strongest not only in the region but in the world, was considered both the symbol and the guarantor of the country's sovereignty and its people's safety.

The army's sitting out the Gulf War did not exactly call this conviction into question, for the means were available and the restraint could be replaced by action if and when it proved disadvantageous. But it did harken uncomfortably back to the days before statehood when the lives of Jews depended on the not-so-good will of others—both of their enemies and of the host of the indifferent who did nothing to staunch the flow of Jewish blood. The callousness of most of the Western world to the plight of the Jews during the Holocaust, with its refusal to believe the grim happenings in time, its curtailment of immigration by Jews fleeing Hitler, and the refusal of England and the United States to bomb the railways carrying Jews to the death camps, all raised doubts, though mostly unvoiced, about just how far Israel could rely on others for its protection.

With this sad history as background, the activities of the Americans on Israel's behalf during the Gulf War were viewed with profound ambivalence. The arrival of the Patriot antimissile batteries after the first attacks on Israel was greeted with relief and appreciation, and the American military personnel who operated them were hailed as saviors of the moment on Israeli television. Similarly, as the damaging attacks on Israel's central coastal region tapered off after the ninth day of the war, the Coalition's search for and destruction of the Scud launchers in western Iraq could be seen to be bringing results.

At the same time, no one could lose sight of the fact that America's interest could and did diverge from Israel's. The Patriots, which the Israeli government had asked for before the war started, were sent in only after Israel was attacked, and the cynical man-in-the-street assessment was that they were sent less to protect Israel than to keep Israel from protecting itself. There was considerable unease about America's continuing refusal to provide Israel with real-time intelligence, a refusal that would have greatly hampered any independent Israeli action in Iraq should the government have considered it necessary. Moreover, there were those who grumbled that Israel's restraint made the country look weak and undermined its deterrent power. As the Scuds continued to land, albeit fewer of them, and as the threat of chemical attack continued to hang over people's heads, the opinion could be heard that the IDF could do a better job of routing out the Scuds than the Coalition air force because it would act more boldly and take more risks. This view perhaps underestimated the complications of such an operation, with the need to fly over Jordanian territory and the risk of pulling Jordan and Iran further into Saddam's camp. But it reflects the very strong feeling that when it comes to the crunch the only ones to defend Israel properly are Israelis; they feel intense discomfort and anxiety when the job is left to others.

The various anxieties converged in connection with the ground war toward the end of February. By this time the Scud attacks had diminished in both frequency and destructiveness. In the last three weeks of February there were only seven strikes, and after the middle of the month none of them did any damage. More than half the people who had fled the scudded area when the missiles began landing had returned, and there was a certain easing of tension and relaxation of vigilance. But Iraqi troops were still in Kuwait, Iraq's much vaunted National Guard was still in place, and the Iraqi dictator was safe in his underground bunker, still in a position to do damage.

The generally agreed-on need for a ground campaign reawakened all the fears and mixed feelings of the days leading up to January 15. On the one hand, there was a good deal of fear that the ground attack would be just the trigger for the still-expected chemical assault. On the other hand, it was feared that the Americans, still traumatized by Vietnam, would not go ahead with it or would withdraw when the casualty count mounted. It was like waiting for a storm: wanting it to clear the air and dreading it at the same time. No one anticipated how easily the Iraqi troops would scatter and the air go out of Saddam's balloon.

The Gulf War ended most appropriately on Purim. This is a boisterous holiday celebrated by masquerade and frolicking that commemorates the rescue of the Jews of ancient Persia from the designs of the evil Haman to exterminate them. For secular and religious Jews alike, the name of Haman is associated with every tyrant who has ever risen up to oppress or injure the Jewish people, and Purim is the holiday that marks the community's salvation. Because of the war, the traditional holiday celebrations were toned down. Parents were warned to keep their kids' costumes simple so that they would not interfere with the donning of gas masks should the need arise; the traditional costume parades in Haifa and Tel Aviv and the other outdoor events that had become centerpieces of the Purim festivities were canceled by orders of the civil defense authorities; and the Purim eve high jinks in which young people walk about town good-naturedly bopping each other and passers-by on the head with light plastic hammers were put on hold. Then came morning, Purim day. The news: the war is over; Saddam surrendered. Israelis left their gas masks at home or in their cars and went out, breathing easier than they had in six weeks, to celebrate, this time for real, the rescue of the Jewish people from the modern-day Haman.

Analogies aside, the intense fear created by the Gulf War will stay with many Israelis for a long time, even though the major threats never materialized. So will the dilemmas they faced as individuals and as a nation. This chapter has tried to describe the general predicament, short-changing in the process many who suffered substantial hardships. The following chapters will focus on the various groups in the population who were affected, each in its own way, by the material damage and persistent uncertainty of the war that was different from every one of Israel's previous wars and that may presage, on its small scale, the face of wars to come.

# 2

# The General Population
## From High Stress to Moderate Habituation

The previous chapter described and explained the fears and stresses of the Gulf War. Its approach was impressionistic, since its aim was, above all, to give the reader a *sense* of what it was like in Israel during the almost six months of waiting for war to break out and the six weeks of waiting for missiles to fall. The rest of the book takes a closer look at the public's response and tries to refine and fill out with hard data the picture drawn thus far. Each chapter focuses on a specific group in the population. Because the Gulf War targeted civilians without regard to gender, age, status, or any other distinguishing feature, we begin our exploration by looking in general at the Israeli public's responses to the war.

## THE PITFALLS OF THE NATURAL LABORATORY

Before we can plunge into our subject, it is necessary to pause to say something about the situation under which the research that forms the basis of this and the following chapters was carried out.

The Gulf War provided a natural laboratory for the study of stress. Usually, the study of stress is either confined to the laboratory or restricted to specific groups of individuals, for example, postpartum mothers, bereaved persons, soldiers, and the like, who experience a given stressor. In the Gulf War, the entire population of Israel was under threat, and both independent researchers and institutions grabbed the opportunity to launch real-time investigations into how Israelis felt, behaved, and perceived the situation. Their studies provide a wealth of information on how a population under threat responds.

On the other hand, the same natural conditions that lend authenticity to human research may lead to finished products riddled with question marks. The problems of the various studies will be pointed out as we go along. Here it is enough to note that most of the studies cited in this chapter—and in the entire book for that matter—were carried out under conditions that gave rise to methodological problems.

It is not only that people's energies were devoted to protecting themselves and their families and getting through the war. It is also that the pressures of the war made it difficult, if not impossible, to plan the studies carefully. The specific circumstances and the issues that were examined often called for improvised measures, whose reliability and validity there was no time to ascertain. Moreover, with little consistency in the measures, it is difficult to compare results and to account properly for the discrepancies that inevitably arise when different researchers look at a phenomenon from different perspectives.

Insufficient time and resources caused other problems as well. The studies carried out by independent researchers tended to use small, unrepresentative samples. The studies undertaken by institutions such as the army and research centers in Israel used large, representative samples, but to question a large number of people under the circumstances of the war, they resorted to the telephone. Telephone surveys can handle only a relatively small number of fairly simple questions. As Klingman, Sagi, and Raviv (1993) state in their discussion of methodological issues, "It became clear that information which can be obtained during war time (mainly self-report and telephone surveys) is limited in scope" (p. 38).

Despite these shortcomings, however, taken together the studies shed light on the public's reactions to the war. Though difficult to compare, their different measures do point to a fairly consistent, two-faceted trend. All of the studies indicate some degree of distress, but, at the same time, they all indicate that for the most part people kept their emotions under control, perceived the situation realistically, and behaved adaptively.

## THE MYTH OF PANIC

In the long prelude to the war, there was widespread apprehension that the threat to the civilian population would lead to mass panic. This apprehensions proved unwarranted, but it was widely held by influential people, including decision makers and mental health professionals. Consequently, it also had repercussions. As a result of this widespread concern, the decision was made to put off the distribution of the gas kits, and the public was instructed not to unpack them or try them out (Omer, 1991). This apprehension may also have been behind some of the hyperactivity of the many mental health professionals who took to the airways and newspapers to calm the public's fears (Granot, 1993) and brought down on themselves a torrent of criticism afterward. The general response to the war is thus of interest not only for purely scientific reasons but also for good, practical ones. There were already indications in the literature that the public's response to the missiles would be more adaptive than the turmoil predicted by the myth.

One line of studies pointing in this direction was on the reactions of people caught up in natural disasters. In his seminal study of human responses to disaster, Drabeck (1986) listed three myths about people's behavior in mass catastrophes: the myth of panic, the myth of looting, and the myth of shock. The first two hold that large-scale catastrophes lead to social disintegration and looting; the third holds that individuals caught up in disasters go into shock, which prevents their responding rationally and requires external intervention. According to Drabeck, none of the myths is true. In disaster after disaster, people kept their heads. Before the disaster struck, they were able to heed warnings, follow instructions, and organize protective measures. During the disaster, both panic and looting were rare. Panic tended to occur only in no-escape situations, where there was an immediate threat to life and people did not know one another; the classic examples are sports stadiums and burning movie houses. Looting, where it happened, was the work of isolated individuals, usually from outside the community. Quarantelli and Dynes (1985) noted the adaptive behavior of people in disasters and even suggested that there were some positive effects.

The other, somewhat limited body of research is closer to home in that it has to do with the responses of civilian populations under attack. One relevant study was carried out by Philip Saigh (1984) on students at the American University of Beirut. Saigh administered three self-report anxiety inventories a month before the 1982 Israeli invasion of Lebanon and then again six months later, after Israeli, Palestinian, and Syrian forces had all withdrawn. He compared the scores of 38 students who had remained in West Beirut throughout the siege with those of another 50 who had evacuated to safe environs. Results showed that the anxiety levels of the two groups were similar both before and after the siege. This suggests that however anxious the students who remained in Beirut might have felt during the war, the shelling did not result in long-term anxiety.

The other pertinent study was an examination by Rachman (1990) of the British psychiatric literature published during World War II, when London was under the German blitz. Rachman tells that before the air raids started, it was generally feared that they would lead to panic. Not only was there no panic, but there were very few psychiatric casualties at all. As he puts it:

> To the considerable surprise of almost everyone, the psychological casualities were few, despite the death and destruction caused by the attacks. Of 578 civilian casualties admitted to hospital in a heavily raided area, only two were suffering primarily from psychological disturbance. A report from another heavily bombed area confirmed that only 15 of the 1100 people treated in medical clinics showed psychological disorders. (p. 20)

Rachman concluded that "rapid *habituation* (adaptation) to the intense stimulation that signaled the imminent appearance of danger is one of the most striking findings to emerge from these experiences" (p. 23).

As consistent as the findings were, however, they were not sufficient to dispel the myth of panic and breakdown in crises. Since the emotional impact of natural disasters is somewhat different from that of disasters created by human beings, it was impossible to know whether the many findings of constructive behavior in earthquakes, accidents, and so forth would apply to the behavior of Israeli civilians threatened by poison gas. The studies of civilians under wartime attack, for their part, were far too few and narrow in scope to serve as foundation for prediction. Rachman's conclusions were based on impressions rather than hard data. And the experimental studies that were carried out on civilians in previous wars in Israel (Hobfoll & London, 1986; Kaffman, 1977; Milgram, 1978; Saffir, Merbaum, Golberg, & Yinon, 1977) focused on issues such as the impact of bereavement and of the father's absence on the family, which were not relevant to the Gulf War, where fathers and sons waited at home for the missiles to strike. Nor could it be assumed that the discipline that Israelis showed in previous wars, which were fought on enemy territory and had few if any civilian casualties, would be practiced when large urban residential areas came under attacks that people could not repulse or defend against.

So the myth persisted even among people of the helping professions who had experience of prior wars in Israel. Shortly before the January 15 ultimatum came due, the Israel Defense Forces' (IDF) Mental Health Department (1991) distributed a document to its medical and mental health personnel warning that "it is expected that many people will be in a state of significant emotional stress" characterized by "feelings of distress and anxiety and by difficulty functioning" (p. 2) and laying down guidelines for treating them.

The studies presented in this chapter relate directly or indirectly to this myth. They focus on people's fear, asking a variety of questions about its intensity, manifestations, and consequences at various points in the war and among various subgroups. We divide the studies roughly (because there is some overlap) into those that surveyed the population in general and those that looked at the relatively small number of Israelis who were treated in the country's general hospitals or who were at special risk.

## PART I: SURVEYS OF THE GENERAL POPULATION

With the missile attacks concentrated in the cities on Israel's coastal plain, most of the population was out of their trajectory; within the target areas, only a small minority were actually exposed to a direct or close hit. Nonetheless, as pointed out in the previous chapter, in the early days of the war people had no way of knowing where the missiles would strike and, later on, even after the pattern had been established, they had no way of knowing that it would not change. For this reason, the threat spread far beyond the physical damage caused by the missile strikes, and tentacles of fear gripped people who were injured in no other way.

Numerous studies were conducted during the war by both public agencies and independent researchers examining the effects of the threat on the general population: on people of all ages and walks of life, who lived with the stresses of the war though they sustained no injuries and their homes were not hit by missiles. Because of their large number, I will present only the most salient and representative studies. For the sake of coherence, I present them in the order that, in my view, best makes their overall point.

## High Morale in Troubled Times

### Three Dimensions of Morale

The first study that I discuss was carried out by Dr. Shlomit Levy of the Louis Guttman Israel Institute of Applied Social Research (1991b). This study examined public morale during the Gulf War in the context of data on morale in Israel collected on a regular basis over the previous 15 years. The surveys were each carried out on representative samples of about 1,200 Jewish adults (age 20 and over), who answered questions in their homes posed by trained interviewers.

As operationalized in this study, public morale consists of three components: instrumental, affective, and cognitive. The instrumental component is assessed by the question "Do you think you can *adjust* to the present situation?" with responses rated on a 4-point scale from "I'm sure I'll be able to" to "I'm sure I won't be able to." The affective component is assessed by the question "How is your *mood* these days?" with responses rated on a 5-point scale, from "good all or almost all the time" to "bad most of the time." The cognitive component is assessed by the question "In your opinion, how is the general situation of Israel today?" with responses rated on a 5-point scale from "very good" to "not at all good."

Figure 2.1 shows the percentage of positive endorsements for each of the dimensions separately. Looking at the graph as a whole, we see that the three dimensions of morale have shown a consistent pattern of relationships over the years, with a relatively high proportion of the respondents (80–90%) endorsing an ability to adjust; a lower proportion, but still more than half (60–70%), endorsing a good mood; and the lowest proportion endorsing a positive assessment of the state of the country. In other words, over the years considerably more people have felt confident in their ability to adjust and have maintained a good mood than have felt positively about the state of affairs in Israel. This pattern applies to the Gulf War as well.

Looking at the three components of the graph separately, one can see a pattern of good morale in troubled times. Of all of the dimensions

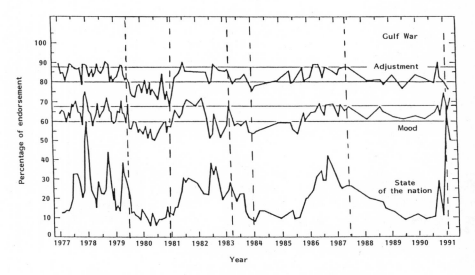

**Figure 2.1.** Morale, mood, and adjustment: Changes over time.

of morale, the only one that seems to have been at all undermined by the Gulf War was people's view of their ability to adjust, and this only slightly. Fewer than 80% of the respondents (70% in Haifa and Tel Aviv, where the missiles landed) reported that they were adjusting well. According to Levy (1991), the dip reflects a transient sense of personal vulnerability. On the other hand, this is not at all a small portion of the population to have felt that they adjusted well to the war's stresses.

The other two dimensions actually show improvement over the years preceding the war. A somewhat higher proportion of respondents reported good mood than over most of the 15 years preceding. This includes the three years of the Intifada (the Palestinian uprising that began in December 1987), when an average 60–70% of Israelis reported good mood, and the time of the Lebanon War (1982–1983) when a relatively modest 50% of the public reported good mood. Levy points out that there is precedent for external difficulties leading to an increase in good mood among Israelis. Citing historical documents on the siege of Jerusalem during the 1948 War of Independence, when the objective conditions under which people lived were extremely difficult, she observes that the harder their lot, the better the public mood.

People's appraisal of the country's situation was also better than in most of the preceding 15 years. In particular, a considerably higher proportion of respondents regarded the country's situation as good than did during the Intifada years. The only time in recent history that more people were optimistic about this was during the Egyptian president Anwar Sadat's visit to Jerusalem in November 1977.

An interesting finding that emerges from this set of comparisons is that public morale, in all three of its aspects, was higher during the Gulf War than during certain periods of peace. In fact, the lowest levels of morale were charted not during wartime but during the peacetime years 1980–1981, when the economy was in deep recession. This suggests that mundane economic strains may have a more deleterious impact on citizens' morale than the life threat of missile attacks.

The picture of personal vulnerability among part of the public along with positive mood and positive assessment of the country's situation relative to the years prior to the war differs, as we will see, in detail from the findings of some of the other studies. As noted above, this is inevitable when different researchers approach the same matter from different perspectives. The overall trend throughout the studies is consistent, however, in that all of them show a mixed reaction, with people displaying signs of distress on the one hand and control and a sense of proportion on the other.

A similar picture is gleaned from another issue investigated by the

Louis Guttman Israel Institute of Applied Social Research: people's nervousness over the years. Subjects were asked "Are you bothered by feelings of nervousness?" at significant dates from 1967 (when the Six Day War was fought) through the end of the Gulf War, and they could reply "frequently," "sometimes," or "never." Findings showed that the rates of people reporting *frequent* nervousness were no higher during the Gulf War (17–19%) than at other times, and were lower than during the 1967 Six Day War (28–29%). Moreover, the number of people who reported that they *never* felt nervous was actually higher during the Gulf War (31–38%) than at other junctures in Israel's history, including during Sadat's peacemaking visit (15%). The incongruity suggests that at least some people may have maintained their morale by denying their nervousness.

## Specific Responses to Stress

The Institute's surveys have the advantage of permitting comparison between reactions during the Gulf War and other times. They have the disadvantage of focusing on general responses rather than on the specific physiological, psychological, and behavioral reactions to stress, either in general or to the Gulf War in particular. The studies that follow concentrate more specifically on these reactions.

### *Sleep*

Since the literature recognizes that sleep disturbances are a common response to stress, Lavie, Carmeli, Mevorach, and Liberman (1991) used two approaches to examine sleep disturbances during the war.

One approach was a telephone survey conducted during the third week of the war of a random sample of 200 men and women from all over Israel. Respondents were asked whether they had difficulties falling asleep and whether they suffered from midsleep awakenings. A total of 28% of those queried complained of one or both types of sleep disturbance. This finding, however, is not as straightforward as it seems. Comparing the responses to those obtained in a 1981 study of Israeli industrial workers, the authors found, on the one hand, that the overall rate of sleep disturbances reported during the war was only slightly higher than those reported 10 years earlier (28% versus 22% in 1981), but that, on the other hand, about four times as many people reported *both* types of disturbances during the Gulf War as did in 1981 (13.5% as compared with 3.4% of those queried). Also of interest was the finding that sleep problems were more prevalent among residents of the areas that sustained missile attacks than among those who lived in other areas, reaching 36.5% in Tel Aviv and 39.1% in Haifa, as opposed to the 28% national average mentioned above. Overall, then, the findings of the survey seem to indicate that the stress of the war created sleep problems in a certain proportion of people and especially for those in the high-risk areas.

The second approach was to assess sleep patterns *objectively* via actigraphic monitoring. The actigraph—a self-contained microcomputer in a small case that is worn strapped to the wrist of the nondominant hand—translates wrist movements, which indicate wakefulness, into an electrical signal that it then records and stores. The rationale for this check was that laboratory studies reveal marked discrepancies between self-reports of sleep problems and actual sleep patterns. Nineteen healthy adult subjects, residents of Tel Aviv and Haifa, who had been studied in this manner previously, wore the actigraphs for seven days, 6 of them between January 22 and January 29 and 13 of them between January 29 and February 2. Results showed that in contrast to the increase in complaints of insomnia, overall objective measures of sleep were only minimally affected. The time it took to fall asleep and the duration and efficiency of sleep (amount of sleep per time spent in bed), during both nights following a missile attack earlier in the evening and nights when there was no such attack, were no different from the quality of sleep of the same people recorded in 1987. The only difference was in their sleep one evening when there was a strike at 1:30 a.m., but even then one subject slept through the alarm and the rest fell asleep again without noticeable carryover.

The authors point out that many insomniacs misperceive their sleep quality. They suggest that many of the people who complained about sleep disturbances in fact suffered only from "fear of sleep," which was provoked by worry that they would sleep through the alarm or that, even if they did hear it, they would be too slow in becoming alert to get into the sealed room or shelter and put on their gas masks in the short time before attack. Rejecting the possibility that the subjects' sleep was affected in a more subtle way than could be detected by the actigraphic recordings (that is, alterations of sleep-stage distribution or intrusion of alpha activity), the authors conclude that these findings may be interpreted as reflecting mainly "environmental insomnia," characterized by *subjective appraisal* of the ability to fall and stay asleep.

The actigraph measurements have the weakness of small sample size as well as the limitations of the device itself. Together, however, the findings of the two approaches suggest that even if people were uneasy and felt that they slept poorly, they did not actually spend their nights in a state of wakefulness that would indicate very major and obtrusive distress. To put it simply, people showed signs of distress, but these were not so serious as to be disruptive in any large measure.

Similar equilibrium is suggested in two other studies that examined the intensity and manifestations of fear among the public.

### Fear in the First Stressful Week of the War

The public's response to the missile attacks during the first stressful week of the war was examined by the Israeli Institute for Military Studies headed by Dr. Reuven Gal (1992). As Gal points out, this was a week of intense uncertainty and high potential danger, when people were first confronted with their lack of control and enforced passivity. Gal sought to investigate how Israelis of different ages and situations reacted to the stress of the repeated Iraqi missile attacks during this week.

To do so, he conducted a telephone survey in two rounds on a convenience sample consisting of four groups of subjects in various proximities to the danger. The first round of the survey was conducted on January 20, following a predawn Scud attack on January 18 and an early morning attack on January 19. The second was conducted four days later on January 24, following attacks on the nights of January 22 and 23. The subjects were divided among (1) residents of greater Tel Aviv, where most of the missiles fell; (2) residents of Haifa, where several missiles fell; (3) permanent residents of Zikhron Ya'akov, a small resort town situated between Tel Aviv and Haifa, where no missiles fell; and (4) wartime visitors to Zikhron Ya'akov, mostly from Tel Aviv, who sought refuge there from the missile attacks and were temporarily staying in a hotel. There were a total of 170 subjects between 17 and 70 years old, of whom 56 participated in both rounds and the rest in one round (39 in the first, 75 in the second).

The study assessed people's fear in its cognitive, emotional, and somatic expressions.

For the cognitive measure, subjects were asked to *appraise* the current situation on a 5-point scale: (1) deathly frightening, (2) very frightening, (3) not so terrible, (4) a challenge, (5) exciting or stimulating. As can be seen from Figure 2.2, the majority of respondents viewed the situation as "not so terrible" or better: a good third regarded it as "very frightening"; but only a very small proportion made the radical assessment of "deathly frightening." In other words, many people believed that there was a good deal to fear, but most seem to have kept a sense of perspective, and only a few seem to have been carried away by their anxieties.

For the emotional measure, the respondents were asked to rate

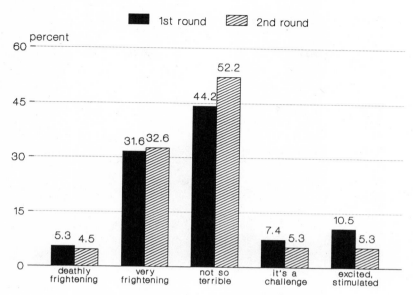

**Figure 2.2.** Percentages reporting different appraisals.

their own fear after the Scud attacks on a 7-point scale from 1 ("I am not afraid at all") to 7 ("I feel strong fear"). In the first round of assessments, administered on the fourth day of the war, the subjects were asked to indicate how afraid they were after each of the first three nights of the war; in the second round, they were asked to indicate only their current level of fear.

Findings showed that, in general, after the first night fear was fairly high, averaging 4.6 on the 7-point scale, but fell to a more moderate 3.6 after the second night and remained relatively constant thereafter. The drop occurred despite the fact that the attack on January 22, two days before the second survey round, caused considerably more damage than the two prior attacks. The first two strikes of the war resulted in minor property damage and a small number of people with light cuts and bruises. In the attack on January 22, six buildings were totaled, three elderly people in the scudded area died of heart attacks, and at least three times as many persons suffered physical injuries. In other words, people seemed to have been getting used to the attacks, even though their threat, at that point, was increasing.

Moreover, as can be seen in Figure 2.3, results also showed that the endorsements differed from group to group. After each of the first three nights, the Tel Avivians endorsed a higher level of fear than any of

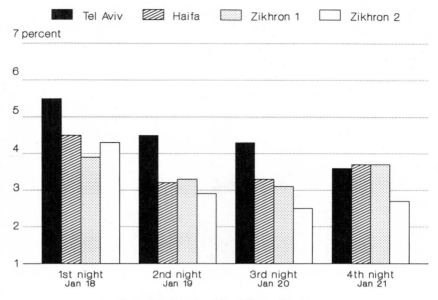

**Figure 2.3.** Fear level by different locations.

the other groups; and, with the exception of the second night, the permanent residents of Zikhron Ya'akov endorsed a lower level.

These differentiated ratings also point to a process of habituation. By January 24, after four missile strikes, the level of fear among the Tel Avivians was no higher than that among the Haifa residents and those who had fled to Zikhron. Within a week of exposure to successive missile strikes, two of them on January 22 and January 23, right before the January 24 assessment, the residents of Tel Aviv were apparently becoming accustomed to the attacks. Those who had fled, on the other hand, were losing their advantage, and in the second assessment they were no less frightened than the people in the scudded cities. We may suggest that they took their fearfulness with them.

In addition to the level of fear, the study also explored its sources. In response to the question "What did you fear most during the air raid?" the clear leader was the uncertainty of the situation, with 41.3% of the respondents in the first round and 51.2% of those in the second naming this factor. Runners-up were fear of chemical attack (32.6% in the first round, going down to 21.3% in the second) and fear of conventional attack (starting at 7.6% in the first round and increasing to 14.2% in the second). In both assessments, more people were afraid of a possible chemical attack than of a conventional strike; at the same time, after four nights of conventional attacks, almost twice as many people named that as their major fear as had in the first assessment. Other sources of fear were hardly mentioned.

Finally, to gauge the expressions of fear, Gal asked subjects to report their most prevalent symptoms in the previous 24 hours. Sleeplessness ranked first (43%), followed by anger and rage (39%), and withdrawal (32%). Gal observes that these symptoms are characteristic responses to helplessness and enforced passivity (Gal & Lazarus, 1975). On the other hand, severe responses such as panic, shortness of breath, weeping, and paralysis were relatively rare (ranging from 15% to 7% of the sample endorsing them). This dichotomy between discomfort and serious upset is consistent with the findings on sleep reported above.

### Comparative Anxiety: Before and during the War

Similar issues were explored in a survey conducted by Hasida Ben-Zur and Moshe Zeidner (1991) of the Wolf Center for Study of Psychological Stress at Haifa University. This study assessed mainly anxiety and bodily symptoms in a convenience sample of 500 respondents, about three-quarters of them residents of Haifa (mean age 34.5). Data collection started at the beginning of the second week of the Gulf War and continued for 31 days, through February 24.

To assess the elevation of anxiety during the war, the authors compared the scores of the above-described "crisis group" (examined during the war) on the 5-item State Anxiety subscale (Zeidner & Ben Zur, 1989) of the Spielberger State-Trait Anxiety Inventory* (Spielberger, Gorsuch, & Lushene, 1970) with the scores of what they term a "norm group" consisting of 409 university students (mean age 23.67) who had participated in a number of research projects in periods of relative peace before the war. As expected, the crisis group reported higher anxiety levels than the comparison group, even when age was controlled for. Moreover, when the responses of the students in the crisis group were isolated and compared with those of the student norm group, the results were almost identical to those for the groups as a whole.

Since the study was conducted over a 31-day period, the authors were also able to examine changes in anxiety and other stress indicators as the war progressed. They did this in two ways: (1) by asking subjects themselves to estimate their level of fear and depression both at the

*The State Anxiety subscale assesses the person's current or transitory emotional state, while the Trait Anxiety subscale examines the way the subject generally feels.

beginning of the war and at the date they filled out the questionnaires on 7-point scales (very low to very high) of these emotions, and (2) by comparing the responses of subjects who filled in the questionnaires at different dates. They found that subjects estimated higher levels of these emotions at the beginning of the crisis than later on when the tests were taken. They also found that the subjects' ratings of their present fear and depression decreased somewhat with the number of days that elapsed since the start of the war. These findings are yet further indications of habituation.

### Steady Accommodation and Persistent Nervousness

The most comprehensive of all the studies was undertaken by the IDF Department of Behavioral Sciences (DBS) and carried out by the staff of its Research Branch: Lieutenant Colonel Avraham Carmeli, Captain Lilach Mevorach, Captain Nira Lieberman, Lieutenant Orit Taubman, Ms. Sigal Kahanovitz, and Professor David Navon. The study consists of 23 surveys of the general population carried out over the entire duration of the prewar and wartime period. The first survey was taken in August 1990, shortly after the Iraqi invasion of Kuwait, and the last one was taken at the end of February 1991, a few days before the announcement of the ceasefire. Eleven were carried out before the war and 12 during.

The purpose of the surveys was to provide the army senior command with information for decision making. The DBS generally gathers data on morale and other such issues *within* the army. But in the Gulf War the battle was on the home front, and many questions arose regarding the civilian population, ranging from whether and when to distribute gas masks to how the public was coping with the war. To answer these questions, it was deemed necessary to query the civilian population.

Data were gathered primarily via nationwide telephone surveys of random samples of adult men and women. Approximately 8,000 subjects participated. Each questionnaire consisted of about 30 items, which varied as the situation changed, with some questions asked in every survey and others asked only as the need arose.

Of all of the studies conducted during or about the Gulf War, this is the most encompassing in scope of inquiry, duration, and number of subjects. Its comprehensiveness and use of a large representative sample give weight to its findings. On the other hand, the reliance on the telephone and the speed with which data had to be gathered, analyzed, and conveyed to the appropriate military bodies resulted in certain confusions. Since it is a very wide-ranging study, I present only selected findings in this chapter, focusing on the overall trend in the public's response to the war. Other findings are discussed in the appropriate chapters.

More specifically, we take a look at three separate but interrelated sets of findings, which can be roughly classed as emotional, cognitive, and behavioral. These findings give a clearer picture of the nature and extent of the habituation noted in the studies cited above.

### Cognitive Responses

The public's perceptions of the threat were gauged by asking their assessments of the likelihood of conventional and nonconventional attacks: In your opinion, how likely is a conventional missile attack on Israel in the near future? In your opinion how likely is a gas missile attack on Israel in the near future?

The data, presented in Figure 2.4, show a number of responses.

First, both before and during the war consistently more people expected conventional than chemical attacks. In August and early September the difference was small, but it became considerably larger after the conventional missiles began to fall. By the end of the war expectations of chemical attack had declined a great deal more than expectations of further conventional strikes. Nonetheless, for most of the war, a quarter of the population continued to expect a chemical attack.

Second, the expectations of both conventional and chemical attack decreased somewhat as the war progressed. This decrease probably reflects the decreased frequency and destructiveness of the actual attacks. Nonetheless, well over half the population continued to expect further attacks of one sort or another to the very last.

Third, their overall decline notwithstanding, the expectancies fluctuated with the actual missile attacks, rising sharply right after each attack and then subsiding a day or two later. However, while expectations of conventional attack continued to fluctuate in this way throughout the war, expectations of chemical attack plateaued by the end of January and did not bound upward with the missile attacks in February.

### Emotional Responses

The public's emotional responses were gauged by their answers to four questions: (1) How apprehensive are you about what might happen to you and your family in case of a *chemical* attack? (2) How apprehensive are you about what might happen to you and your family in case of a *conventional* missile attack? (3) In your opinion, how panicky are the people around you? (4) How worried are you about the country's securi-

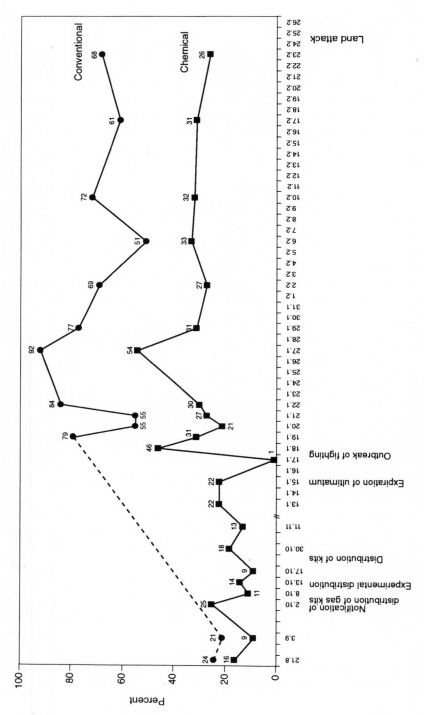

**Figure 2.4.** Expectations of missile attack.

ty situation? These questions were answered on a 5-point scale ranging from very little to very much. The percentages of people who endorsed the highest two levels on each of the three questions are presented in Figures 2.5 and 2.6.

As can be seen, the curves of the four emotional responses are fairly similar in shape. For the most part, when people were apprehensive about the possible damage of a conventional attack, they also were apprehensive about the possible damage of a chemical attack, were worried about the country's security situation, and reported more panic around them than when they were less apprehensive. Moreover, the curves are also roughly similar to the pattern of expectations of conventional attack. These parallelisms are logical, because all the emotional questions similarly tap anxiety about the threat and because such anxiety would naturally coincide with the expectations of the threat being realized.

More telling, the graph points to the coexistence of two diverse trends: emotional accommodation and persistent nervousness.

*Accommodation.* As the war progressed and as fewer people expected further attack, the public's emotional reactions to the war decreased in intensity. The reduction can be seen in two ways. First, the percentage of people who reported feeling strong fear *in between the missile attacks* gradually declined: fewer people reported great apprehension about the consequences of a conventional attack, and fewer people reported great worry about the country's security situation. The decline occurred despite the destruction of people's homes in the missile strikes, but might reflect the fact that few people were seriously injured or killed. Second, as the war progressed, fewer and fewer people reported strong fear *in the wake of each attack*. In February, fewer people endorsed great apprehension about the consequences of possible conventional attack immediately following each strike than had in January; fewer reported seeing panic in others; and fewer reported strong concern with the security situation. The authors of the report term the overall downward trend "habituation" and the decline in the percentage of people responding intensely to each missile attack "minihabituation." In their terms, there was a dual process of habituation and minihabituation.

*Nervousness.* The other trend is that people remained on edge. This too can be seen in several ways. For one thing, the data point to the persistence and strength of Israelis' fears of chemical attack, despite their decreased expectations of it and even as conventional warheads were flattening their homes. Although their between-strike apprehension about the consequences of a possible conventional strike declined in

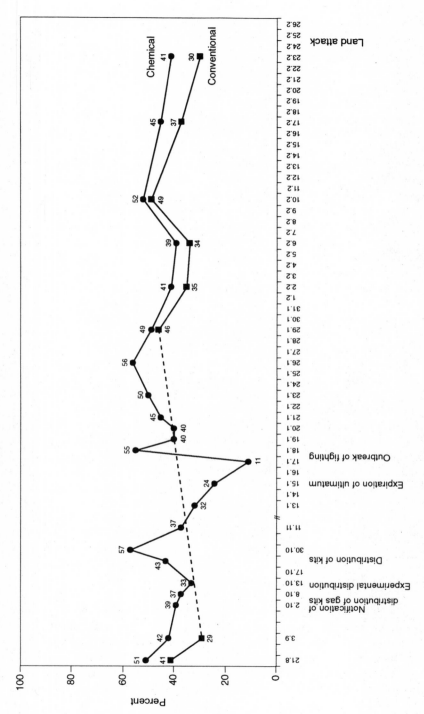

**Figure 2.5.** Apprehension about the results of chemical and conventional attacks.

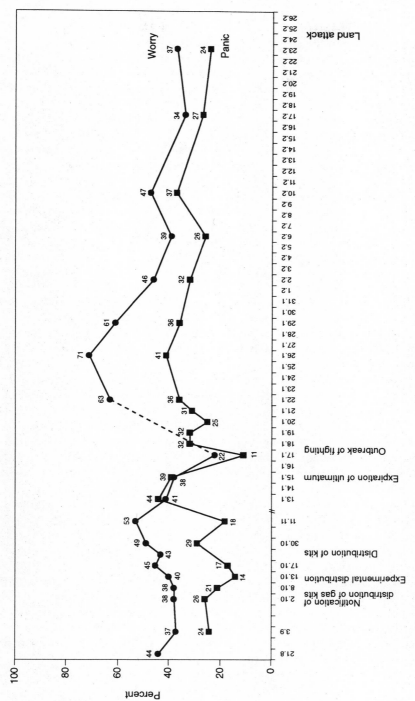

**Figure 2.6.** Worry and panic.

the course of the war, their apprehension of the consequences of a chemical strike did not. In the surveys taken on January 19 and 20, 40% of those queried endorsed great apprehension of the consequences of a chemical attack; in the last survey of the war, taken on February 24, great apprehension was endorsed by 41%. Moreover, throughout most of the prewar and wartime periods, about 10% more of the population endorsed great apprehension of the possible outcome of a chemical attack than endorsed such apprehension about the consequences of a conventional one. The difference is relatively small, but it is fairly consistent and telling.

The other clear indication of persistent nervousness is in the upward jump in the level of fear with every reminder of the danger, whether actual or symbolic. Before the war, intense anxiety about the damage of both chemical and conventional attacks was most pervasive right after Iraq's invasion of Kuwait and at the time the gas kits were distributed, an event that confirmed the danger and forced it into people's awareness. At the outbreak of the war, public anxiety plummeted briefly with the Coalition invasion of Iraq, only to shoot up sharply with the first missile attack, when it became clear that the invasion would not work an instant miracle. But after that, anxiety fluctuated throughout the war, rising steeply after every major missile strike, after people were injured and homes destroyed.

The fluctuations in observed panic were pretty much the same, with one notable difference. The high point was just before the expiration of the Coalition ultimatum, when 39–44% of those queried reported that people around them were in a state of panic, though the self-reports of anxiety were not particularly high then. It is possible to conjecture that the unprecedented and highly publicized flight of Israelis abroad at this time was both an expression of and a contributor to the widespread *sense* of panic.

Concern about the security situation followed a similar pattern, with the one exception being that the gas mask distribution seems to have calmed, rather than intensified, people's fears in that respect. (Incidently, the percentage of respondents who endorsed high concern about the country's security situation was lower than the percentage who endorsed high fear on the other measures. This relationship is inconsistent with the finding in the Louis Guttman Israel Institute of Applied Social Research study (Levy, S., 1991b), cited above, of a relatively low proportion of respondents expressing optimism about the country's security situation. The discrepancy may be rooted in the different ways in which the question was phrased in the two studies.)

To be sure, these sharp increases in the percentages of people who endorsed strong fear were very brief, lasting for only about a day or so before a new equilibrium was established at a lower level of fear and the trend of accommodation was resumed. However, the lability of the responses suggests that a good portion of Israelis had an underlying reservoir of fear that they apparently kept in check but that surfaced when the danger was thrust into their awareness. In other words, it seems that a certain proportion of people who were generally able to control their fear and endorsed only moderate levels in the surveys (the report does not provide percentages) could no longer do so when the missiles struck.

Yet another indication of underlying fear kept under control is the difference in the public's cognitive and emotional endorsements. Throughout the war a considerably higher proportion of those surveyed reported that they expected further attacks than admitted being apprehensive of the consequences, worried about the country's security situation, or witnesses to signs of panic in others. This discrepancy suggests that more people may have been ready to admit to cognizance of the danger than to fear of it. It suggests that fear existed but was not always acknowledged and (like the findings of low levels of nervousness in the Louis Guttman Israel Institute of Applied Social Research ([Levy, S., 1991b] study cited above) that a good portion of the population used denial to contain their anxiety and maintain their spirit.

### Behavioral Responses

The public's behavioral responses were ascertained in a number of ways. The two most direct ones were assessment of somatic symptoms and coping.

*Somatic Symptoms in the Sealed Room.* The findings again show a pattern of intense anxiety early in the war followed by increasing accommodation. When asked whether they had experienced any unusual bodily sensations while in the sealed room (burning sensations, tears, breathing difficulties, trembling, excessive perspiration, or any others), a substantial 38% answered in the affirmative at the first inquiry on January 18, but by the second inquiry a day later their number was down to 27% and slumped even further to only 18% and 20% in the second and third weeks of the war.

*Coping.* People were asked to rate their coping with the war on a 4-point scale. Findings show that as their anxiety and somatic complaints decreased, people's self-assessments of their coping increased. At the end of January, 73% answered that they coped well or very well (the top two levels); by the last week of February, 90% reported that they coped well or very well. Moreover, various groups in the population (that is, persons over age 51, the poorly educated) who had reported relatively poor coping in January reported coping as well or almost as well as the better copers by the end of the war.

The coping pattern of the people in the greater Tel Aviv area, where most of the Scuds struck, was somewhat different. Throughout much of the war, substantially smaller proportions of Tel Avivians than people living elsewhere reported that they were coping well or very well. Furthermore, while for most of the public the sense of mastery improved steadily in the course of the war and was unaffected by the missile strikes, this was not the case for the Tel Avivians. Their sense of coping was particularly poor in the surveys taken soon after missile strikes, suggesting the impact of the attacks in the people most subject to them. All the same, however, even in the Tel Aviv area, at least two-thirds of the respondents reported good or very good coping throughout. This is not a small proportion considering the immediate threat to life and property they were under.

These data show that people were affected by but nonetheless managed to cope with the difficulties of the war. They are consistent with the findings discussed above of the Louis Guttman Israel Institute of Applied Social Research that almost 80% of their respondents felt confident of their ability to adjust to the situation at hand.

In short, these two assessments show an appreciable decrease in somatic complaints and a concomitant increase in perceived mastery as people came to expect fewer attacks and became somewhat habituated emotionally. Moreover, the fluctuations that characterized people's emotional and cognitive responses were generally absent from their behavioral ones. On the whole their somatic complaints did not saunter upward and their sense of mastery did not plunge downward with every missile attack. The difference suggests that even while a substantial proportion of people continued to feel worry and fear, they were soon able to get a grip on the behavioral manifestations of their distress. People apparently learned to cope with the threat and to live adaptively while continuing to experience relatively high levels of fear. The partial exception, as pointed out above, were the residents of the greater Tel Aviv area, whose sense of mastery was undermined somewhat by the missile attacks.

Two other behavioral assessments fill out the picture of how Israelis responded to the war. One is of people's compliance with the emergency instructions; the other is of the Israelis who left their homes in search of safer parts of the country.

*Compliance with Emergency Instructions.* To ascertain the extent to which the population followed those instructions, the study asked three questions: Will you go into your sealed room/shelter at the next alarm? Do you always take your gas kit with you when you leave your home? During the last alarm, did you wear your gas mask until you were told you could remove it?

Results show that almost all Israelis took—or said they would take—shelter during the alarms (97–85%); a smaller but still substantial proportion took their gas kits with them when they left their homes (87–57%); and the smallest proportion, but still the majority, wore their gas masks until the army spokesman announced they could be removed (77–57%). To be sure, there was never full compliance. Even in the high-risk areas, and more so outside of them, a small number of individuals failed to take shelter and to wear their gas masks altogether, while others left the shelters and removed their masks before instructions to do so were issued. Moreover, compliance with all the instructions decreased somewhat in February, though the only substantial reduction was in the proportion of respondents who kept their gas masks on for the full duration required.

These lapses notwithstanding, on the whole the indications are that the public followed instructions and behaved in a disciplined manner. Considering the circumstances, the rate of compliance was fairly high. It is not really surprising that after a while people outside the stricken areas would become lax. Nor should it be surprising that after the sealed rooms proved ineffective protection against the conventional missiles and the chemical threat failed to materialize, at least some people would feel that the safety measures were not worth the trouble and take other actions.

The protective measure least observed was wearing the gas mask. The authors suggest that this reflected genuine difficulties. Confirmation for this hypothesis is obtained in their finding that 28% of adults and around double that percentage of children reported difficulties in wearing their gas masks. The difficulties included breathing problems, discomfort, and, among young children, fear of the masks and refusal to put them on.

Further confirmation is provided by other professionals. The psychiatrist Dr. Moshe Isaac pointed out in a newspaper interview in January (Namir, 1991) that the masks caused some people to feel a sense of helplessness and suffocation. Medical complications associated with the gas mask, including transient hypoxia, especially in persons with cardio-pulmonary disorders, were reported by a group of physicians at the Beilinson Medical Center (Huminer, Pitlik, Katz, Metzker, & David,

1991). Also reported were hyperventilation, gastrointestinal symptoms, exacerbation of asthma and angina (Borkan & Reis, 1991), and dermatological complications of various sorts resulting from the vacuum created by the well-sealed mask (Vardy, Laver, Zakai-Rones, & Klaus, 1991; Zimran & Ashkenazi, 1991).

*Leaving Home.* As noted in the previous chapter, large numbers of people left Israel just before the war started. When the missiles began to strike, even more left their homes for safer parts of the country. The DBS attempted to assess their number, their sociodemographic and personal characteristics, and whether their leaving helped them cope.

Given the limitations of a telephone survey, the number of departees could be assessed only indirectly, by asking respondents how many apartments there were in their building and how many of their neighbors had left, and then calculating the percentage of empty apartments and using this to estimate the number of people not living in their homes at any given point in time. On this basis, the researchers estimated that 34% of the residents of the greater Tel Aviv area had left their homes, for a greater or lesser amount of time, in contrast to only 3% in other parts of the country.

Because of the difficulty of locating those who left, their characteristics and coping were measured in a one-time assessment the last week of the war (February 24–25), when most people had returned to their homes. At that time, the researchers interviewed a sample of Tel Aviv residents, consisting of both those who had stayed and those who had left.

Their findings show that the groups were quite similar in a fair number of ways. They were similarly apprehensive about the effects of a possible chemical or conventional missile attack, made similar assessments of their children's anxiety levels, and reported similar levels of faith in the IDF and similar levels of agreement with the government's policy of restraint.

They differed, however, in both sociodemographic features and what might be interpreted as their fearfulness or cautiousness. With regard to the first, they tended to be younger and better educated than those who stayed, and more of them had children under age two. In other words, they were evidently more able to leave and had more incentive to do so.

With regard to the second, more of those who left than those who stayed were worried about the country's security situation, perceived panic in the people around them, and felt stress after dark, when the Scuds struck. They also exhibited more caution in their compliance with the safety instructions: a higher proportion of them wore their gas masks during the missile alarms, a higher proportion took their gas masks along outside their homes, and a higher proportion went down to the shelters (instead of into the sealed room in their apartments), presumably in search of greater safety, when an alarm sounded.

Their self-assessed coping levels, on the other hand, were similarly high: 85% of those who had left and 92% of those who had stayed said they were coping well. The researchers concluded that leaving the high-risk area did not give those who did so any advantage over those who stayed. Their findings are consistent with those of the Institute for Military Studies (Gal, 1992), which showed that the people who left Tel Aviv for the resort town of Zikhron Ya'akov soon lost any advantage in peace of mind their flight may initially have given them. On the other hand, those who left may have had more to cope with or, as the authors suggest, lower coping levels than the others to begin with, in which case their flight from the danger zone could be regarded as an adaptive act. The lack of comparative data on their coping before and after they left makes it difficult to judge the benefits of their departure. Another interpretation of the findings is that any difference in the coping of the two groups would have disappeared by the end of the war, when most people felt less threatened and were coping better than they had been earlier on.

### Trust in the Country and Its Institutions

Taken together, the findings of the DBS study point to two simultaneous responses.

On the one hand, the population responded to the war in a well-disciplined, self-controlled manner. Most people kept their anxieties under control, followed the emergency instructions, and maintained their sense of mastery under attack. Those who had difficulty coping with the attacks can be said to have acted adaptively in leaving the high-risk zone. Extreme responses—from serious somatic complaints to counterphobic disregard of instructions—were relatively rare. Moreover, as the war progressed, fewer and fewer people responded with high anxiety, despite continuing expectation of attack: fewer people reported strong emotional responses, somatic complaints decreased, and sense of mastery increased.

On the other hand, signs of nervousness persisted throughout the war. The enduring nervousness was most evident in the upward leap in the percentage of people endorsing strong emotional responses right after every missile attack. Nervousness is also suggested in the continuing expectation of attack as well as in the fact that consistently more people said that they expected further attack than endorsed strong apprehension about the consequences.

Potentially, either of these trends can be emphasized. One can say with equal justification that people adjusted despite their anxieties and that they remained nervous despite their self-control. In fact, it could be said that both statements are true, and both are required for a full picture.

The high level of coping during the war may perhaps be explained by yet another set of findings in the report. Among its assessments, the DBS also measured Israelis' trust in the country's leadership and policies. It found that throughout the war, a very high proportion of the population (87–99%) retained faith in the army's ability to defend the country from a conventional attack. The DBS also found that a good portion (71–96%) trusted the army spokesman, and that well over the majority supported the government's policy of restraint (79–91%).

The trust was maintained despite the fact that the army did not prevent or retaliate against the missile strikes and despite the fact, too, that many people were skeptical of the value of the protective devices (only 70% gave a positive endorsement). The high agreement and trust point to the continuing confidence of Israelis in their society and, by extension, in themselves, as well as to their continuing identification with the country and its institutions. It may be suggested that at least for those who stayed in Israel and were there to answer the telephone, the identification and confidence ran deeper than the manifold stresses of the war and helped to see them through.

## PART II: THE CASUALTIES

The overall adaptation notwithstanding, the Gulf War, like other wars, did have its psychological casualties. Like the behavior of the general public, these too were assessed by both institutions and independent researchers.

### Hospital Admissions

Basic information on hospital admissions was obtained from three bodies: Israel's Ministry of Health; the Kupat Holim Health Fund, the country's major provider of health care; and the IDF Medical Corps. These bodies work in concert to plan and administer emergency health services during wartime. The country's succession of frequent wars gave rise to a tradition of real-time systematic assessment of wartime needs, parallel to the assessments of psychological needs made by the army's DBS. The Gulf War was no exception. Throughout the war, rates and types of casualties were systematically assessed.

Throughout the war, the IDF Medical Corps collected data on all emergency admissions to 12 major hospitals during the first eight hours after each missile alarm, whether there was an actual missile attack or not (Kersenty et al., 1991). All in all, there were 1,059 war-related hospital emergency room admissions. Two hundred thirty-four of them were what the authors term *direct casualties* (that is, people whose injuries were a direct outcome of the missile strikes), and 825 were *indirect casualties* (that is, people whose injuries could not be attributed directly to damage caused by the missiles).

Of the 234 direct casualties, an overwhelming majority, 221 suffered only mild injuries; 10 sustained moderate injuries (mostly orthopedic); 1 (a three-year-old girl) was severely injured; and 2 were killed in the explosions. Interviews conducted with 39% ($N$=91) of these casualties (the authors tell that many of those who were lightly injured went home before the interviewers reached the hospitals) revealed that 22.2% suffered no physical injury at all but were in a state of acute psychological distress.

The 825 indirect casualties, among them people who arrived in the emergency rooms after five false alarms, were about three-and-a-half times as numerous as the direct ones and counted more fatalities. These casualties consisted of 11 people who died, 4 of heart attacks, 7 of suffocation by gas masks that were worn with their airtight caps on; 40 people who hurt themselves while rushing to safety at the sound of the alarm; 230 persons who needlessly injected themselves with atropin (the nerve-gas antidote that was distributed with the gas kits); and a hefty 544 patients who were admitted with symptoms of acute psychological distress.

These figures show the toll of fear. They show that more people died of fear than of the missile strikes themselves. They further show that large numbers of people, including those who lived in areas where the missiles did not land at all, had accidents that can be at least partly attributed to fear or were anxious enough to feel that they needed medical help. The figures also indicate that as many as 70% of all the casualties (if the "false" atropin injections are included) were psychological in nature.

At the same time, however, further analysis of the data reveals that the same process of accommodation that was documented among the general population operated in the treated population as well. Examining the figures on atropin self-injection, the authors of the study report that there were progressively fewer such self-injections in the course of the war.

Similarly, a study by Bleich and colleagues (Bleich, Dycian, Koslovsky, Solomon, & Weiner, 1992), using the same data, which examined the pattern of the emergency room referrals for stress reaction and self-injection of atropin over time, found that most of these admissions followed the first missile attack and that the numbers dropped sharply thereafter. As can be seen in Figure 2.7, the second missile attack brought only about a quarter the number of psychological casualties as the first, even though that strike caused more physical damage; by the seventh attack the psychological casualties could be counted on the fingers of one hand; and from the twelfth strike on, a few fingers of one hand did quite nicely.

## Referrals to Hospital Social Services

Similar patterns emerge from inspection of the wartime referrals of emergency room patients to the social services at the Sheba Medical Center, Israel's largest medical complex, located outside Tel Aviv adjacent to an area that sustained a fair number of missile attacks.

The authors found that between January 16 and February 26, medical personnel referred 141 people in the emergency room to social work-

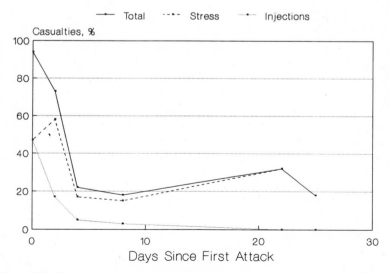

**Figure 2.7.** Stress reactions and injections since first attack for six missile attacks.

ers, in contrast to only 5 persons in the same period the previous year. They were referred with a range of problems, including several that were special to the war situation: loss of housing, difficulty finding family members, fear of being alone, and fear for their lives. According to the authors, the large increase may have reflected either the massive trauma that this population underwent or the high visibility and accessibility of the social workers, or both. They point out that during the war, social workers were in round-the-clock physical attendance in the emergency room, though ordinarily they are only on call but not actually present.

Here too the data show that the majority of the referrals were not direct casualties of the missile attacks. Classifying the referrals into four groups, the authors found that only 39% of the total were *direct casualties,* who were evacuated to the hospital immediately after their homes were damaged or destroyed by missiles and whose symptoms stemmed directly from that experience. Another 28% were what the social workers termed *definite indirect casualties,* who arrived at the hospital a short time after an attack with physical or psychological complaints stemming from the war even though they sustained no bodily wounds and their homes had not been hit. Twenty percent were *probable indirect casualties,* who arrived at the emergency ward anywhere from a few hours to a few days after a missile attack with problems that they themselves did not connect with the war but the social workers did. Only 13% were *casualties not related to the war,* who presented with problems that neither they nor the social workers considered to be related to the war. This classification is consistent with the findings of the Medical Corps' study (Kersenty et al., 1991) that most of the wartime casualties were *indirect,* and it provides yet further evidence of the power of the threat to upset people who were not injured directly by the missiles.

At the same time, the study also supports the accommodation shown in the Medical Corps' investigations (Bleich et al., 1992; Kersenty et al., 1991). It found that 59% of the referrals arrived in January, during the first two weeks of the war, as opposed to only 41% in almost the entire month of February.

## Mortality

Adversity has consistently been implicated in promoting mortality (for example, Holmes & Rahe, 1967). A study of mortality rates during the war carried out by a team of epidemiologists from the IDF and the Ministry of Health (Danenberg et al., 1991) showed the ability of the population to "tolerate a subacute period of psychological stress without excess mortality" (p. 630). Monitoring daily death counts, the researchers found that the population-adjusted mortality rate in the second half of January 1991 and in February 1991 was *lower* than that of the comparable months of the preceding decade, 1981–1990, with which they compared it. Furthermore, they found that the wartime and prewar death rates were not substantially different even in the scudded greater Tel Aviv area.

## Cardiac Patients

At the same time, certain segments of the population seem to have been particularly vulnerable to the stress of the war. As noted above, there were 11 fatalities resulting from heart failure and/or suffocation during or shortly after the missile attacks. The literature (Hinkle, 1974; Holmes & Rahe, 1967) gives reason to believe that such deaths can result from stress. Two studies bear out the suspicion that cardiac patients were at particular risk in the Gulf War.

### Soroka Hospital

A study conducted in the coronary outpatient clinic of the Soroka Hospital in the Negev (Israel's southern region) aimed to assess the effects of the Gulf War on ischemic heart disease patients, who were found to be at high risk for sudden deterioration of their health status during and after the missile attacks. The authors distributed questionnaires to 100 cardiac outpatients during the last week of the war, which tapped their responses during three different stages of the war: the week before the outbreak of fighting, when the perceived threat was on the rise; the first week of the war, when tensions peaked as the threat was actualized in missile attacks; and the last week of the war, when the perception of threat had abated and the atmosphere in the country had relaxed. Three types of patient reactions were assessed: psychological (for example, worry that the excitement of the war might cause heart problems), physical (anginal pains), and behavioral (for example, medication consumption).

Results showed that the intensity of all responses increased significantly between the week before the war and the first, stressful week after the fighting started. In the last week of the war, however, when the perceived threat was significantly reduced, the intensity of the patients' worry decreased, but there was no concomitant reduction in frequency of anginal pains or in medicine consumption.

The researchers postulated that there may be two distinct processes of adjustment—psychological and physical—and that while people react promptly to threat alleviation on a psychological level, their physical adaptation is delayed. They argue that the persistence of the relatively high frequency of physical symptoms after the perceived threat and concerns that may have caused them had diminished supports the life events model to the effect that exposure to stress may result in long-term deleterious physical effects. They further suggest that the persistence of more frequent anginal pain might point to the irreversibility of the damage of the war to the physical condition of coronary patients.

## Meir Hospital

Doctors at the Meir General Hospital in Kfar Saba (Meisel et al., 1991) examined the incidence of acute myocardial infarction (MI) and sudden death in a catchment area in the center of Israel that covers 400,000 people. Rates of MI were examined in the first week of the Gulf War (January 17–24, 1991) and were then contrasted with two earlier periods: two weeks in January and two weeks in July of the previous year. Results showed that in the first week of the war there was almost a threefold increase in the incidence of acute MI and almost a twofold increase in rates of sudden death outside the hospital. The doctors also found that there was a disproportionately high increase in acute *anterior* MI. After the first week of the war, no further increases in rates of MI or sudden death were found. The authors maintain that not only the anxiety and terror aroused by the missiles, but also the gas masks, may have contributed to ischemia by reducing airflow, causing a cycle of fright, ischemia, and possible reduction in oxygen supply.

Both these studies suggest something of the damage that the stresses of the war did to cardiac patients. And while both point to some degree of accommodation, the findings at Soroka indicate that the adjustment may have been superficial and that, in fact, the war did cause these patients long-term harm.

## CONCLUSIONS

The studies discussed in this chapter are substantially different from one another. They use different measures, examine different parts of the population and by different means, and to some extent focus on different periods of the war. Nonetheless, taken together, their findings all point in the same direction. They show that on the whole Israelis coped adaptively with the stresses of the war.

To be sure, all of the studies reveal some degree of distress, whether in terms of perceived ability to adjust, self-reported sleep difficulties and other somatic complaints, heightened anxiety, and fear at the time of the missile strikes or apprehension about their consequences. They show the difficulty of living with the uncertainties of the situation and the persistent fear of chemical attack. They also show that the Tel Avivians in the center of the storm felt less a sense of mastery than people on the periphery. Moreover, the data on hospital admissions indicate that, as in other wars, there were psychiatric casualties and even fatalities that could be attributed to stress.

At the same time, extensive evidence of adaptation stands side by side with the evidence of distress. Most people contained their fears and maintained their equilibrium. Relatively few people expressed fears that were out of bounds. Most people observed the emergency instructions and retained their confidence in the country's leaders and defense establishment. The somatic symptoms they had, including their sleep disturbances, were neither paralyzing nor even highly disruptive. The psychiatric casualties who arrived at the hospital emergency rooms and social services were not so numerous as to impose a burden. The major sufferers as a group were cardiac patients, who are known to be at high risk under stressful circumstances. Some of them can be said to have died of fear, some due to faulty use of the masks, but otherwise there was no increase in mortality.

Moreover, from the very beginning of the war a process of accommodation began. By the end of the first week, people were calmer than they had been at the beginning; by the end of February, fewer people displayed strong anxiety than had in January. As the war went on, levels of depression declined, fewer people reported somatic symptoms of fear, and more and more people indicated that they felt a sense of mastery and ability to cope. These adjustments occurred despite the fact that the missile threat remained and even though many people continued to expect further missile attacks to the very end of the war.

Although each of the studies presented in this chapter has its limitations, they combine to provide a coherent, though diverse, picture of people's conduct during a national crisis. This picture is remarkably close to that drawn by Rachman (1990) of the British under the German blitz. Though the times and circumstances were quite different, and Israelis were not subjected to anything near the long, constant bombings to which Rachman's Londoners were, the behaviors of the two populations can be described in similar terms: neither has a substantial number of psychiatric casualties, and both became rapidly habituated to the stress. The virtue of the above studies on the Gulf War is that they provide empirical, real-time evidence for what Rachman concluded almost 50 years after the event on the basis of impressions gathered from a review of the psychiatric literature.

These studies should thus contribute to dispelling the still-pervasive myth that people behave irrationally in large public disasters and that both ego control and the social fabric disintegrate. On the contrary. The studies provide no reason for concern that substantial numbers of Israelis—with the possible exception of people who lost their homes in the missile strikes (to be discussed later on in this book)—will suffer posttraumatic effects from the Gulf War.

Nor is there any evidence for the disruption of the social order. Perhaps the most important conclusion of the studies was that, for all its anxiety, the public behaved rationally throughout. Though respondents in the IDF's DBS study reported that they observed panic in people around them, that panic was limited. There are reasons to believe that these observations referred to the sight of neighbors leaving the country and, later on, the Tel Aviv area. We may suggest that these observations may also have referred to outbursts of temper, displays of tension, hyperactivity, and people worrying about themselves and one another. But at no point was there any behavior that can be described as mass panic. In the early days of the war, there was some hoarding, mainly of baking soda, which was supposed to help in the case of chemical poisoning, and staples such as bread and milk. But these can be considered rational, protective measures. There was no rioting, no looting, and no vast disregard for other people's rights and safety.

Indeed, the society continued to function within the limitations imposed by the emergency routine. After the first four days of the war, people went back to their jobs. Shops remained open during the day. Eventually the schools were reopened, with parents helping to monitor them. In apartment buildings, neighbors got together to seal their common shelter and stayed in it together. The buses ran. Hospitals had emergency plans and were staffed by doctors and nurses doing 24-hour duty. Volunteers offered their help in all sorts of tasks, from serving the aged to assisting the people displaced in the missile attacks. And social scientists planned and carried out the studies that cannot possibly capture the enterprise and vitality of the population as it kept going despite the ever-present threat.

# 3

# Forced Intimacy
## The Israeli Family in the Gulf War

Families are usually divided during wartime: men leave for the front; women and children stay behind. There are letters, phone calls, worry and longing, the struggle to cope without the husband/father/bread-winner, and all the complex emotions attendant on separation and then return. In the Gulf War, where missiles struck at civilian targets, the home was quite literally the front. The family was tested not by distance and the absence of its male head but by prolonged enforced togetherness —by what Dr. Ze'ev Bergman (1991) of the Jerusalem Family Clinic has termed "forced intimacy."

The intimacy was naturally concentrated in the nuclear family. With the notable and numerous exception of families in which the man stayed in a high-risk area, usually to go on with his work, while the woman and children sought refuge in a safer part of the country, most families spent an inordinate amount of time cooped up together at home. We already noted that schools were shut for the first three weeks of the war, so that many children spent the better part of their day at home, often with their mothers. But even in families where both parents worked and continued to work during the war, come sundown everyone was back together under the same roof—and stayed there. Gone were the occasional evenings out, the Friday-night visits with friends or relatives, the cup of coffee at the neighborhood café, the movie, play, concert, folk-dancing night, or bridge with the pals. Gone were all the activities that break the routine of work, supper, and sleep; that bring adults into contact with their peers; and that husbands and wives can enjoy together or separately, but that in any case introduce interest and variety into their relationship and diffuse the potentially trying intensity of constant one-to-one contact.

From the nuclear family, the enforced intimacy in many cases spread to the extended family and even friends. People fleeing the targeted areas sought shelter with whoever could provide it elsewhere: parents, siblings, cousins, uncles and aunts, old school or army friends— anyone who was out of the line of fire and had an open door. With their bags and kids, they packed into their hosts' generally small homes already brimming over with their own family members. Some people came together for other reasons too: ex-spouses moved back with each other for the sake of the kids, elderly parents came to be taken care of by their adult children, or adult children who had long been living on their own returned to the parental home.

Crowded together in apartments whose size tends to match the Lilliputian dimensions of the country and deprived of their usual social, recreational, and occupational outlets, supports, and avenues of expression, family members could have a hard time carving out and maintaining the personal space from which they could then interact and support one another. In the family, the balance of togetherness and separateness, of closeness and distance, was inevitably upset.

Symbolically, the repeated sojourns in the sealed room may be regarded as the epitome of the intense togetherness and all its pressures. The typical room might have been anything from 10 to 15 square feet, enough space for a man and his wife or a few children, but not for more. With the windows covered and taped, and with the door shut and taped up after everyone was inside, the room could be claustrophobic. At the sound of the alarm, everyone who was in the house or apartment crowded into the sealed room. Everyone had to find a space, as long as it was not against a wall with a window or opposite a wall with a window. Everyone had to cooperate, or anything could go wrong: A slowpoke who did not manage to get into the room quickly could prevent the others from taping the door shut in time; a child or an older person who needed help with his or her mask might not get it. The very conditions that made efficiency and cooperation so necessary could mitigate against them. Moreover, whatever prior tensions were present in the family and whatever emotions the family members harbored—fear, frustration, anger—were inevitably brought into the room and sealed into it with the occupants.

But the difficulties were not confined to the sealed room. The underlying tension and fear in which most people lived during the war and the pressing conditions the war created tried people's tempers and self-control. The war upset the routines that make for the smooth operation of the household and that, to some extent, govern people's interactions. In many homes, dinner and bedtime preparations were pushed up so that family members would not be caught at the table or in the shower during an alarm. Among other things, this could make for a rush on the bathrooms. In some homes, children slept in their parents' bedroom, either for a sense of security or because it had been made the sealed room. In yet other homes, children who ordinarily played outside or visited friends freely stayed at home for considerable periods, idle, bored, and under foot.

The special situation called for a reallocation of roles in the family and put to the test the family's ability to respond with flexibility to changing conditions. At the same time, the close confines and mutual dependency of family members on one another could provide the setting and incentive for the social support that, as is well known, reduces stress and helps people cope in crises. The forced intimacy doubtless created pressures, but it could be serviceable as well.

Existing knowledge provided little indication of how families would actually deal with the pressures of the war or what impact those pressures might have on them. Family stress theory originally developed out of the study of the dynamics of families where the husband/father was away at war (Boss, McCubbin, & Lester, 1979; Hill, 1949; McCubbin & Patterson, 1983). There are very few studies of the impact of war itself on the family unit. The studies relate mainly to families of soldiers, especially to those of MIAs and POWs, and concentrate on such matters as the effects on the family of separation from the soldier (father, husband, son): fear for the soldier's safety, the postwar reunion (for example, Hunter, 1978), and the soldier's death or injury. More recently, the impact of the returning soldier's posttraumatic stress disorder (PTSD) on his family has received scientific attention (for example, Solomon, 1988). None of these issues is relevant to the Gulf War, and there are no studies, to our knowledge, of the effects of war per se on the family as such.

With two exceptions, there are, as far as we know, no systematic studies of Israeli families in the Gulf War either, even though other segments of the population—soldiers, children, and elderly people, to mention only a few examples—have been investigated. We can conjecture that the absence of a theoretical framework, the shortness of the conflict, and the particularly complicated logistics of family research, in which ideally all members of the family should be examined, all played a role.

In the remainder of this chapter we present the limited information that is available, focusing on the ways in which Israeli families coped with the hardships of the war and on the impact the war had on them. We begin with the two studies just mentioned and go on the personal testimonies and clinical reports.

## FAMILY SOLIDARITY

One of the areas explored in the survey conducted by the Israel Defense Forces' (IDF) Department of Behavioral Sciences (described in Chapter 2) was the impact of the Gulf War on family relations. In a telephone survey, subjects were asked how the war affected their family life and were presented with choices ranging from "positively" to "not at all" to "negatively."

Results showed that most respondents, 56%, felt that the emergency situation and the subsequent changes in routine did not affect their family at all; 38% felt that it improved their family life; and only 6% felt that it damaged family relationships.

Men and women perceived the impact similarly, as did respondents living close to where the missiles struck and those living farther away. On the other hand, a larger percentage of older respondents (70% of those age 51 and over) than younger ones (52% of the 26- to 40-year-olds and 45% of the 41- to 50-year-olds) felt that the war did not affect their family relationships either for better or for worse. It can be suggested that either their relationships were more solid by that time in their lives, so less subject to strain, or that, not having small children, they had fewer war pressures with which to cope. Education also moderated the impact of the war: the more schooling, the less the impact. Of respondents with an elementary school education, 48% reported no effect, as opposed to 56% of those with a high school education and 61% of those with higher education. Moreover, more respondents with higher education (45%) reported that the war had a positive effect on their family life than respondents with a high school education (39%), and more of them reported a positive impact than those with only an elementary school education (33%). This is consistent with other findings on the ability of education to moderate stress.

Family relationships in this study were examined along with the impact of the war on other areas of functioning, namely, work, economic situation, and daily routine. Of all these areas, family life seemed to be the least affected, and most of the changes that were reported were for the better. This means that most Israeli families coped well with the pressures of the war. We know from the literature that external threats generally lead to greater affiliation and solidarity among people (for example, Cohen & Dotan, 1976). This study shows that the cohesion of

Israeli families during the war was stronger than the pressures driving family members apart.

## STRESSES ON THE FAMILY AND FAMILY FUNCTIONING

Other than the above, the only other systematic study we know of that explored the direct impact of the war on Israel's families (Ben-David & Lavee, 1992; Lavee & Ben-David, 1993) was conducted by Yoav Lavee and Amit Ben-David of the Center for Research and Study of the Family at the School of Social Work at Haifa University. The study, which was carried out between January 21 and 24, 1991, a few days into the first week of the war, focuses on family perceptions and functioning during the air raids.

Sixty-six families were randomly selected from a telephone directory of the greater Haifa area, which sustained several direct missile hits just before and during the time of the study. In each family, a semistructured telephone interview was conducted with the adult family member who answered the phone. Forty-three (65%) of the respondents were wives, 19 (29%) were husbands, and 4 (6%) were adult children living with their parents. Of the families contacted, 55 (83%) had children under the age of 18 living with them. The rest were older couples with children living elsewhere.

The interviewer posed open-ended questions focused on the time between the sound of the alarm and the release from the sealed room. Families were found to differ in four areas: (1) perception of the stresses of the war and missile attacks, (2) perception of the threat, (3) family interaction when the alarm went off and in the sealed room, and (4) current and predicted impact of the war on the family.

Four *sources of stress* were delineated:

1. Existential life fear, as expressed, for example, in the statement "The missile will fall right here on us and we'll die."
2. The war's numerous ambiguities and uncertainties, especially whether the missiles had chemical warheads and the resultant quandary of whether to go to the sealed room or to the bomb shelter when the siren sounded. Other uncertainties included the fear of not hearing the alarm in time to take cover and the question of how long the war would last and how it would end.
3. Hardships associated with the war, including the protracted stay at home, the bother of getting up at night, the crowding in the sealed room, and difficulties breathing through the gas masks.
4. Intrafamily strains arising from the circumstances of the war or

from prior tensions exacerbated by the war. The authors suggest that a major strain was the need to change ways of coping with closeness and distance. They illustrate the point with two telling quotations: "The home is like a pressure cooker . . . there's no way to let the steam out. My husband is used to working long hours, and all of a sudden he had to stay at home" and "The children are at home all day long for too long . . . they get on each other's nerves and our nerves too."

Families differed in how many of these stressors they reported—though most reported more than one—and in the relative salience of the stressors. Unfortunately, there is no statistical examination of either the frequency or the level of the stressors.

Similarly, four *perceptions of the situation* are delineated. These are that the situation is:

1. *Catastrophic*—an assessment that tended to be accompanied by intense existential fear and to include the idea that the war could develop into a cataclysmic worldwide crisis.
2. *Terrible*—that the war is much more difficult than expected and will go on for a long time.
3. *Difficult and frightening*—but it could be worse and might even have some long-term benefits.
4. *Bearable*—especially in comparison with previous wars. Respondents were relieved that the war was being fought outside of Israel and "our boys aren't fighting it."

Again, frequencies are not presented.

Family *patterns of interaction* in the sealed room were ranged along three dimensions:

1. *Emotional atmosphere* was characterized by various combinations of fear and security. The authors divide the families into those that expressed fear (high anxiety) and those that expressed a sense of safety (low anxiety). They then divide both groups once again. Among the fearful were families practically overwhelmed with terror when the alarm sounded ("It was like a nightmare. . . . I don't even remember very clearly anymore. We were shaking and frightened. We thought that if we didn't put our masks on, we'd die") and families who were afraid of the missiles but confident that their masks and sealed room would protect them. Among the secure families were those who took comfort in the low probability of a missile falling just where they lived, on the one end of the spectrum, and, on the other end, those who were shielded from anxiety by their fatalism. As one respondent put it,

"What will be, will be. . . . There's nothing we can do to protect ourselves anyway."

2. *Mode of family organization* referred to the distribution of tasks in
going into and being in the sealed room. Here too families could be
divided into two groups: those in which family members had distinct,
well-defined tasks (for example, the father sealed the door while the
mother helped the kids on with their masks) and those in which there
was no such allocation of duties and anyone who happened to be nearby
would turn off the heating and lights or get the dog. Although they do
not actually say so, the authors imply that the latter mode of organization was inefficient and confusing, with lights that were switched off and
on and with family members who did not quite know what to do in the
sealed room.

3. *Interpersonal interaction* in the sealed room varied quantitatively
and qualitatively. Quantitatively, some families reported being in constant interaction—talking, laughing, and taking pictures of each other
with the gas masks on—while others reported minimal exchange—
reading, listening to the radio, or engaging in silent contemplation.
Qualitatively, the interaction could be positive or negative, with conversation and exchange of ideas and jokes, on the one hand, or quarreling
and shouting, on the other. As this family tells, "We fought with the kids
about putting on their masks, and also between ourselves about whether
the kids should put on their masks. There was a lot of yelling and noise."
The same held for noninteraction. In some families, the noninteraction
was calm and supportive. Family members sat quietly, ruminating, reading, or clustered around the radio or television, respectful of one another's space and need for distance. In other families, the noninteraction
was alienated and tense. As one young woman described it, "Mother sat
on the bed and didn't say a word. Father was also very quiet, but it was
clear that he wanted to leave the room, which he actually did before the
all-clear sounded. I'd taken a game into the room, one of those puzzle
cubes, and played by myself. I was not very successful though."

For the *current and predicted impact of the war on the family,* three major
response combinations emerged:

1. *Positive–neutral:* the belief that the imposed closeness was bringing the family together and making it closer for the time being
   but was unlikely to have any lasting impact.
2. *Neutral–positive:* the view that the imposed togetherness had no
   current effect on the family but would strengthen it in the long
   term. These were families who were accustomed to spending

time together before the war. As one respondent put it, "We are a
family that spends a lot of time together. I've read in the paper
that some families bless the opportunity to be together at last. We
didn't have that surprise."

3. *Negative–neutral:* the feeling that the compulsory togetherness
and confinement were oppressive and suffocating but would not
have any long-term impact on their family.

Among the most interesting aspects of the study are the portraits
that the authors draw of four family types. Though they present different parts of the picture in each of their two papers (Ben-David & Lavee,
1992; Lavee & Ben-David, 1993), for economy and coherence we merge
them. The four family types the authors name are anxious, cautions,
secure, and indifferent.

*Anxious families* were most troubled by the external stresses of the
war—by the threat of death, destruction, and annihilation. They expressed fears that they would be struck by a Scud, that their homes
would collapse on them, and that nothing would protect them from the
poison gas. They tended to perceive the situation as catastrophic. They
also reported considerable intrafamily strains, derived from their intense and freely expresssed anxiety as well from differences among
family members in their perception of the threat. The fear and interpersonal conflict exacerbated one another.

Anxious families were unable to organize themselves effectively in
going into the sealed room, and once they were inside, there was quarreling, shouting, and confusion as to who would do what. Nonetheless,
these same families voiced positive feelings about being together and
regarded the forced intimacy as good for them, even if they did not
expect it to have any long-term effect.

*Cautious families* reported experiencing all four types of stressors:
life fear, uncertainty, war-related hardships, and intrafamily strains. The
authors attribute this inclusiveness to the openness of cautious families'
communication, which allowed them to vent all their feelings (but the
authors do not explain why equally expressive anxious families reported
a smaller range). These families tended to perceive the war as "terrible,"
only a grade less serious than the "catastrophic" assessment of the anxious families.

The most salient difference between cautious and anxious families
was in their conduct in the sealed room. Despite their anxiety, cautious
families were well organized, with each family member knowing what to
do and doing it. Moreover, their interpersonal interaction in the room
was marked by mutual support, discussion of problems (for example,

what to do if a family member had to go to the bathroom), and the use of humor. This was considerably more functional than the quarreling of the anxious family. At the same time, their assessments of the impact of the war on their families was similar to those of the anxious family: the enforced family togetherness was beneficial but unlikely to have any lasting impact.

*Secure families'* major sources of stress were the war's ambiguities and uncertainties. Most often, these families expressed concern about not knowing how the situation would develop, what to expect, and what to do. They also complained about the inconvenience of getting up in the middle of the night, the discomfort of the gas masks, and the difficulty of not being able to go out freely or let their children out. Whatever anxiety they might have felt was kept in check by their sense of the statistical improbability—to which they frequently referred—of a missile striking just where they happened to be. They tended to perceive the war as difficult but not as bad as it might have been and to be optimistic about the future.

When the alarms sounded, these families were more relaxed than anxious or cautious families, and were able to manage the threat in a cooperative way. Roles were clearly allocated, and there was a definite sense that the family unit was able to organize itself and work effectively to protect its members. Their interaction in the sealed room was less intense than that of anxious or cautious families, and family members tended to be preoccupied each with his or her own thoughts, but in their quiet, nonverbal way they did seem to provide each other with mutual support. In considering the impact of the war, respondents from secure families expressed the view that the compulsory togetherness had no immediate effect but that the shared experience would strengthen the family bond in the long term.

*Indifferent families* typically claimed there was nothing stressful about the war and expressed neither fear nor any other overt emotion. When pressed, they conceded that dealing with the children was not easy, but added that since they were calm, their kids were too. They tended to see the war as a positive event that would eliminate the Iraqi threat and make peace in the region possible. They regarded the situation as quite bearable and preferable to the prewar waiting period.

At the sound of the alarm, some of them did not go into the sealed room. Among those who did, there was no clear-cut division of labor, and once inside there was little interaction but a great deal of tension, which tended to be absorbed by the children. In some indifferent families, one or more family members left the sealed room before the all-clear was given. These families reported that the war, especially the confinement at home and in the sealed room, was not a good experience for the family. Evidently they found the togetherness excessive. They did not, however, expect any lasting effect on the family.

Although the authors do not say so, one may guess that at least some portion of the "indifferent" families were denying the threat and suppressing their anxiety, which then surfaced in the tension in the sealed room or was transferred to the children. It is also possible to regard the refusal to go into the sealed room and the early departure from it as counterphobic measures. Alternatively, it may reflect a belief that the damage was so great that the sealed room was an inappropriate protective measure.

As noted above, aside from the IDF survey, this investigation is the only study to focus on the interesting and important topic of family functioning during the Gulf War. As a qualitative investigation, it is also the only study to attempt to grapple with the complexities of how families coped with the war. Nonetheless, the study is highly preliminary.

Its major drawback, which the IDF study discussed above also has, is that only one member of each family was interviewed. Though the authors insist that they repeatedly asked whether the respondents' views were shared by other family members, it remains that only one view was obtained, and there is no way of knowing how representative that view really was. In the next chapter, the differences in the responses of men and women to the Gulf War suggest that there may well have been less agreement than the authors' presentation implies. In my view, the family portraits are too monolithic, and any interplay or clash of opinions among family members gets short shrift. Divided families—that is, families in which the members may not have all found the same things stressful, perceived the threat in the same manner, judged the family interaction similarly, and felt that the war had the same impact on the family—are conspicuously absent. From my own limited experience, I know that in more than a few families, one adult tended to express all the existential fears while the other denied or disregarded them and was bothered by the disruption in routine and other inconveniences.

A second problem is the lack of even basic quantitative information. While qualitative description sheds light on family functioning in a way that statistics do not, it would be valuable and interesting to know, for example, what proportion of families perceived what stresses and what proportion belonged to each type. Furthermore, analysis of the relationships among the variable might have, among other things, shed light on the conditions under which external threat leads to cohesion and those under which it leads to disruption, as well as on the relative probabilities of these outcomes.

Nonetheless, the study does indicate the large variety of responses to the war and the range of ways that families dealt with its many pressures. It is unrealistic to expect flawless methodology in a study carried out in the midst of a crisis. The authors themselves point out that the timing of the study, the first week of the war, made it impossible for them to assess the war's long-term impact and that therefore they had to be content with people's predictions of what that would be. But the timing also had considerable advantage. The study was carried out when popular anxiety was at its peak, as we saw in Chapter 2, and also when the four-day "curfew" at the outbreak of the war, in which workplaces were shut and people advised to stay at home, was still fresh in memory. This made it possible to tap the immediate responses to what were among the war's major characteristics: fear and imposed intimacy.

Indeed, some of the findings of the study are consistent with observations made by Ofra Ayalon (1991) of the University of Haifa in a paper on the effects of the Gulf War on the civilian population. The coping strategies she observed among individuals who defined themselves as "good copers" with the war—especially the strategies of taking comfort in the small probability of a missile striking their exact location, having confidence in the gas masks and the sealed room, and keeping in mind that Israel had weathered greater dangers in the past—are much the same as the strategies Lavee and Ben-David (1993) found among families whose anxiety level was low. She also observes that the "forced intimacy" could have different implications and consequences, depending on the family's prewar interactions (that is, the intimacy could provide a sense of comfort and security or produce feelings of suffocation leading to aggression and conflict) (Ayalon, 1983; Ayalon & Zimrin, 1990).

## FORCED INTIMACY VERSUS FAMILY COHESIVENESS

We now turn to the various personal testimonies and clinical reports that came out of the war. These present a variety of effects, both positive and negative. The commonly accepted view is that crises intensify or bring to the surface whatever strengths or problems the family already has. According to Bergman (1991), the Gulf War "magnified and intensified processes that already existed in the family." Zivit Abramson, head of the family therapy unit at the Adler Institute, elaborated on the view in a newspaper interview conducted in early February 1991: "Nothing happened unexpectedly; it just seemed as if new and different things were occurring. Actually, things were just as they had been before;

people just weren't aware of them. Families found themselves in positive and negative situations. . . . On the one hand, intolerable friction, tension, and pressures in addition to war-related anxieties; on the other hand, outbursts of warmth and closeness. These are not changes. The new conditions . . . brought to the surface hidden processes" (Shaked, 1991). Although this supposition has never been tested empirically, it is behind much of the case material available to us.

Bergman (1991) suggests that reactions to the war varied with the family's stage of development and the couple's relationship. Using a modified version of Bergman's scheme, we present some of the interpersonal issues raised by the war and alternative responses of family members to it. Since much of the information we have derives from clinical sources, there is perhaps too much emphasis on the problem that surfaced with the war. It should be kept in mind, however, that in no small number of families the war brought out the best in the individual members and revealed their capacity to work together and support one another in time of need.

## THE COUPLE RELATIONSHIP

The forced intimacy and role changes of the war pushed some couples apart and brought others together.

### Overturning the Applecart

The following account, published in a daily newspaper (Shaked, 1991), illustrates how the conditions of the war revealed the underlying emptiness and strains of what had seemed to the woman of the house, a mother and schoolteacher, a harmonious family life. As becomes apparent in her testimony, the harmony was superficial and had depended on the husband's working late and on the couple's sharp traditional gender division of labor and authority. The underlying stresses surfaced when the war kept the husband at home and he became involved in the household management:

> The war, which forced us to spend so much time at home with the children, turned our life into a nightmare. Suddenly I saw that the harmony that had existed was external and superficial, the product of years of routine and our interaction. My husband works in a management job and usually comes home late in the evening. I work part-time and spend most of my time at home. The house, which had always been my territory, suddenly became our joint domain. He's become impossible. He gets into my hair, has begun to criticize how I run the house; he tries to teach me how to cook the soup; he's angry that I don't iron all the clothes; he'll take the

garbage down only in the morning. . . . Up until the war, I was the one in charge of all household matters. Now the kids don't know who to turn to. They talk to me, then they go to their father out of respect, and get contradictory instructions. This family, which I was so proud of, suddenly looks like a house of cards.

Bergman (1991) suggests that the midlife families most susceptible to disruption on account of the role changes fostered by the war were those that had not till then achieved an adequate balance between partners. As an example, he describes a traditional couple with rigid role divisions, not unlike those in the above account. The man was a successful professional and the woman a housewife. At the outbreak of the war the husband's elderly parents came to live with them. The husband became anxious and stopped going to work. The wife became a volunteer in the emergency services, where she spent long hours, and continued to care for the household when she got home. The husband, neither supporting nor protecting his family, felt divested of his masculine functions and went into a depression. The wife became the center of the family and flourished. The more she flourished the deeper grew her husband's depression.

In the first example, the husband, forced to stay at home, infringed on his wife's autonomy and authority in an area that she had considered all her own and that traditionally is held to be the woman's domain. In the second, the husband who stayed home of his own volition lost the sense of masculine identity that comes from working, and he grew increasingly envious and withdrawn as his wife developed her own personality. In both cases, the change in roles and routines revealed underlying flaws in the couple's relationship and threatened to undermine the marriage.

According to Bergman, the balance the couple achieves in the course of their marriage cements their relationship and is the basis for their intimacy. The war, he claims, increased people's need for closeness, and husbands and wives who had not achieved intimacy felt frightened and alone and looked harder for it. The intense need could either drive the final wedge between estranged spouses or bring them together. As an example of the first, Bergman tells of a couple in their forties whose relationship had long been distant. The wife, who for years had combined a yearning for closeness with a sense of inferiority to her husband, felt rejected when he spent his time at home sealing the room and readying the house for war rather than interacting with her, and she began to discuss separation. As an example of the second, Bergman presents another man and woman in their forties who had been in marital therapy for a long time because of tensions created by the husband's infidelities, among other things. When the war broke out, the couple was at the end of therapy, and the long stay at home provided the opportunity for intimacy for which they were now ready.

**New Perspectives**

The Lavee and Ben-David (1993) study discussed earlier documented both conflict and cooperation in family coping with the stresses of the war. It is generally accepted that cooperation in a common endeavor can bring people together and make them feel closer to one another. An interview conducted during the war with a man and woman who had separated four months before the war on the wife's initiative, after years of quarreling and futile attempts at reconciliation, illustrates this point (Shaked, 1991). On the second day of the war, the wife phoned her estranged husband:

> Suddenly everything changed in my mind. The most important thing for me was the children's well-being, and I understood that it would be very difficult to take care of them on my own. I told him: "I think that we have a common interest and now is the time to unite around it." He agreed and was back home in an hour with his suitcase. We experienced during the first ten days of the war what we hadn't known our entire marriage. We suddenly became the best of friends. The barriers, the arguments, and the legal tug of war that had filled our heads just two weeks earlier suddenly all became irrelevant. Before, the way he ate would drive me crazy; now all of a sudden I didn't even notice it. I don't know why.
>
> It's great. He caught me in the kitchen, spontaneously, with a real big hug. His whole attitude toward me has completely changed. Suddenly his habit of falling asleep in front of the TV doesn't bother me either. Today, I even enjoy falling asleep next to him on the couch. He's suddenly able to play with the children for hours on the floor, doing a puzzle. He can actually do the shopping on his own without a list from me. Even our sex life is better. It's warm and giving.

The external threat seems to have altered the proportions of things, dwarfing irritants that once seemed important and changing the couple's perspective. Their common purpose—to take care of their children in the crisis—and their recognition of their need for one another evidently gave this couple an improved appreciation of each another and increased their empathy and acceptance. As the husband describes it:

> I suddenly found myself in her shoes. The war gave me the chance to see what a load she carried. I realized how much she took care of the children. How much time she devotes to them and how capable she is.
>
> We didn't spend much time together in the past. Now she's open and uninhibited. It's suddenly easy to understand things, easy to appreciate her, easy to sense and feel her.

These instances illustrate only some of the many permutations the war effected in the couple relationship, bringing to the surface latent tensions, on the one hand, and allowing couples to rediscover one another, on the other.

## TEMPORARY SEPARATIONS

If the war kept unhappy families temporarily together, it pushed other families apart, especially families living in the high-risk areas. In these areas, many women took the children and moved in with friends and relatives in parts of the country less prone to missile attack, or even abroad, while their husbands stayed on in the danger zone. We don't have figures, but the phenomenon was widely reported, and everyone knew of people who did it. The reason commonly given for thus splitting the family was that the woman and children could enjoy greater safety, while the man had to stay behind to go to work.

But security was not the only motive. Some women left because it was easier for both them and their kids to be where the children could play outside and did not have to stay indoors for hours and days on end. There were also men who were relieved to have their anxious wife and kids out of the way, in which case the arrangement reflected the difference in the husband's and wife's perceptions of the danger. As we will see in the next chapter, men tended to assess the situation as less dangerous than did women.

Depending on the motive and background, the temporary separation could ease the pressure of the intense togetherness enforced by the war or could reflect or lead to a family rift (Lev-Ari & Bostan, 1991) if the man left in the danger zone felt he was being abandoned or if the woman who departed for greener fields resented her husband's not coming along. In either case, one or both members of the couple apparently felt better being apart during the war than together. As we discuss more fully below, people tend to seek affiliation in times of crisis. Couples who separated evidently did not find the same comfort and support in each other's presence as did couples who voluntarily stayed together.

## THE TRANSGENERATIONAL FAMILY: PARENTS AND CHILDREN, CHILDREN AND PARENTS

Just as the Gulf War tested the couple relationship, it also put to the test the cohesion and functioning of the transgenerational family, consisting of children, parents, and grandparents. As we point out in other chapters, both children and the elderly had their own particular problems during the war. It was left to the middle generation, the caretaking generation, who had children of their own and were themselves grown children of aging parents, to mediate the hurdles for both. This section will deal with the issue facing the vertical family during the war from the point of view of the middle generation.

### The Challenge: A New Order for Young Children

For families with young children, the war, especially the first three weeks when the schools were shut, was somewhat like a boring summer vacation, only much worse. The usual diversions—the outings to the beach and park, visits to museums, trips to the matinee—were all out of bounds. The Scouts didn't meet; the music, arts and crafts, and sports groups that Israeli children tend to frequent were suspended; and the community centers where many activities are held were closed. In ordinary times, even very young children in Israel, from about five and up, are permitted to play outside without parental supervision and to visit friends on their own. With the danger of the Scuds, these freedoms were suspended. Unless they were old enough and able enough to put their mask on and seal the room by themselves, children could not be left alone, even at home while their mothers went to the supermarket. Thus, children were left with few outlets for their energy, while a parent or other adult had to be constantly around just in case. The restrictions were somewhat eased as the war went on and no Scuds landed in the daytime, but they were never totally lifted.

One challenge for parents was keeping their kids constructively occupied after they had become satiated with television. A related challenge was providing an alternative structure to school, homework, afternoon activities, and bed at a certain hour, or whatever routine each family had before the war. The war disrupted children's routines as much as it did those of adults, if not more. One of the major disruptions was the interruption of sleep by the nighttime missile attacks, sometimes several in one night. Some families who could tried to ease these interruptions by turning the children's room into the sealed room or by making their own bedroom the sealed room and having their children sleep with them there. Even so, the nighttime air raids left many children, and their parents too, tired and strung out the morning after. The tiredness, in turn, could exacerbate the children's boredom and whatever anxiety they felt on their own or absorbed from their parents.

The various disruptions reopened issues of household order. Even where there were clear rules before the war, parents had to tackle anew questions like, How late should children be allowed to stay up at night? How late should they be permitted to sleep in the morning? How much television should they be allowed to watch? How should their fears be handled? Should frightened children be allowed to sleep with their parents? Should children be accompanied to the toilet? Should they be supervised while they played? On the answers to such and other seemingly trivial questions, the order of the household depended.

New rules had to be worked out that took into consideration the demands of the war and the emotional pressures it created. Parents were asked to provide their children with emotional support while establishing clear boundaries and standards of conduct, to calm and make allowances for their children's anxiety, and to obtain their cooperation both inside and outside the sealed rooms. To do so, parents had to be able to control their tempers, in many cases frayed by the anxieties and tensions of the war, and to keep their own fears in check.

If they could not juggle all these demands, and if they had not established clear boundaries before the war, they could find themselves with wild, difficult-to-control boys and girls. Bergman (1991), for example, tells of a couple who had been in counseling with him to help them set boundaries for their eight-year-old and five-year-old. When the war broke out, the couple felt that the children were under enough pressure as it was and were reluctant to discipline them. The children went out of control altogether. Less extreme versions of this scenario were played out in many homes where the parents were not able to create a sense of order to replace the routines and structures disrupted by the war. In such homes, bored, anxious children tested limits; parents, tense themselves and wary of adding to the war's pressures, were reluctant or unable to enforce them; and there was a general sense of conflict and disarray.

In families that were more orderly and cohesive to begin with, the war brought out the maturity of the children and their willingness to cooperate. A newspaper article published during the war (Shaked, 1991) observes that "[m]any parents . . . suddenly discovered that they [their children] are little adults, who can be counted on and are sweet and pleasant and helpful, ready to share in the household chores" (pp. 7–8). The writer attributes the responsibility that these children showed to the opportunity the war gave them to express their best selves and to the sense of involvement and family cohesion it promoted.

## Adolescents: Individuals in Their Own Right

Adolescents were more mobile, able to make freer choices, and less dependent on their parents than were their younger siblings. They could organize their time by themselves, and they did not need their parents to mediate the war for them. At the same time, the forced intimacy of the war was precisely the type of situation to exacerbate the major dilemma of adolescence: finding a balance between the need for attachment to family and parents and the need to break away and assert one's own individuality.

In families where that balance was difficult to come by, the war could provide a convenient occasion for adolescent rebellion or push the introverted adolescent further into himself or herself. As an example of the first, Bergman (1991) tells of an adolescent girl living with her divorced mother who used the outbreak of the war to play on the conflict between her parents and move in with her father, who lived in a more dangerous area. In illustration of the second, Bergman presents the case of a 15-year-old who had not been permitted to form his own separate identity. As a child, he had filled the emotional vacuum that his father, an ambitious man who rarely expressed his feelings, had left in his mother's life. As the boy grew up and felt the need to develop his own identity, he lost patience with his mother, defined rigid boundaries between himself and both parents, and fiercely guarded his privacy. Then, during the war, both sets of grandparents came to stay with the family, while his parents projected their anxiety onto him. In reaction to the physical and emotional crowding, the young man withdrew even further into himself.

On the other hand, in families that encouraged it, the war provided adolescents with the opportunity to express their individuality in a mature and constructive manner. Ordinarily, Israeli families make relatively few demands on their children, adolescents included, to help out or take on responsibilities at home. The prevailing mind-set is that childhood in Israel ends abruptly with military induction at age 18 and a hard adulthood follows, so kids should be allowed to be kids. But, during the war, that assumption was suspended and, at least in some homes, adolescents, who could seal the room, take care of their younger siblings, and so forth, were considered material to the safety and smooth running of the household; they were expected to contribute no less than adults, and they did. In one area in particular, adolescents could be most instrumental. We noted in Chapter 1 that the gas mask training for the civilian population was superficial and that people were not given the opportunity to try on their masks or practice using them before the war. The big exception were schoolchildren. Especially during the first air raids, older children and adolescents were in a position to help their parents.

In their book on divorce, Wallerstein and Blakeslee (1989) observe that the crisis of their parents' breakup turned some rebellious adolescents into responsible, cooperative individuals who helped carry the family through the difficult process. Although no studies have been done, I suspect that much the same can be said of many adolescents in the Gulf War. I know that in my own family, my then 11-year-old son and

12-year-old daughter were models of maturity and responsibility. They took care of their four-year-old cousin who had come to live with us and of their grandmother as well. When my mother took ill and neither I nor my husband were in the house, it was they who called the ambulance.

## CARING FOR ELDERLY PARENTS

Although many elderly people were left to fend for themselves during the war, others moved in with their children and grandchildren for all or part of the period. Some moved in because they needed assistance getting into the sealed room, putting on their masks, and taping up the door with the necessary speed and dexterity. Others moved in because they could not, or were afraid they would not be able to, hear the alarm or understand the instructions that came over the radio, or because they could not cope simultaneously with the exigencies of the war and the ailments of old age. Yet others were loath to be on their own in a time of crisis.

For the grown children who took them in, it was an opportunity to return some of the care that their parents had once given them. Yet even among those who accepted the responsibility as right and natural, and where all the people involved got on well, the joining of the generations during the war could give rise to conflict.

The circumstances of the war created two particular types of difficulty beyond all the interpersonal conflicts that can develop when the generations live together. One had to do with the fact that it could be as problematic leaving an elderly parent alone to deal with a possible alarm as it was a young child. This further restricted the already limited mobility of the middle generation. For example, a mother who could not leave her children alone could still get out occasionally by taking them with her as long as she brought along their gas masks. In case of an air raid, children could run or be carried. But with an elderly person or persons to mind, even that little room for maneuver was curtailed.

The other difficulty was that caring for parents could create conflicts of responsibility in a life-threatening situation. For example, who should be helped on with their gas mask first—Grandma or five-year-old Eli? And what should be done if Grandpa can't be gotten into the sealed room before the boom goes off? Should the children's and everyone else's safety be put at risk? Such dilemmas were most pronounced in families with small children, but could arise even in homes where the children had grown up or left if the middle generation themselves felt endangered.

It does not take much imagination to grasp the mixture of resentment and guilt that could grow out of either or both sets of difficulties.

## GOING VISITING

As previously stated, many people living in the high-risk zones moved in with friends and relatives in parts of the country less prone to missile attack. In all probability, this clustering was motivated not only by concern for safety but also by the desire for affiliation. In a laboratory study, Schacter (1959) has shown that people who were rendered highly anxious had a stronger desire to be with others than did people who were less anxious. Applying this finding, Cohen and Dotan (1976) suggested that the coming together of families that occurred during the 1973 Yom Kippur War in Israel was motivated by the wish for affiliation provoked by the war anxieties.

The clustering could have two effects. Where people had a good relationship and refrained from impinging too much on one another's space, it could bring a feeling of comfort and security. For example, Bergman (1991) presents two sisters who had always gotten on well who moved in together after one of their husbands was mobilized. To ensure peace in close quarters, they laid down a number of ground rules: avoid criticism, especially about the behavior of each other's kids; do not impose chores on the other—all the adults agreed to set chores they didn't mind doing; keep everyone, both young and old, occupied; and make sure that the adults had some time for themselves, without the children, even if only late at night. Toward the end of the war, the mobilized husband was released from military duty and joined the extended family. Both sisters and their husbands told that being together significantly alleviated their anxiety and sense of isolation in the dangerous situation. They parted with more than a little regret.

Where the ingredients for harmony were missing, however, the close physical proximity could lead to dissatisfaction and tension. A case in point is a woman I know of who took her three-and-a-half-year-old son and moved in with her brother and sister-in-law and their four kids in Beer Sheva, in the south of Israel. Because she lived in Ramat Gan, the area of the major Scud damage, she sought a safe shelter more than company. She and her sister-in-law could hardly have been more different. One was orderly and organized; the other left things about wherever they fell. One wanted the kids washed and in bed by eight or nine; the other let them lie fully clothed in front of the television until sleep overcame them. One felt acutely uncomfortable with the lack of structure; the other resented the unspoken criticism. The children were disoriented, as much by the interpersonal tension as by the war, and they were ornery. The men kept their distance. The guest felt unwelcome, and her hostess felt intruded on. Everyone was relieved to go his or her own way when the time came.

## PEOPLE ON THEIR OWN

Although this chapter concentrates on the stresses of the war on families, the war was also very difficult, perhaps even more so, for people living on their own: both singles and noncustodial divorcees.

It should not take much imagination to realize how awful it could be to sit by oneself in the sealed room, gas mask on one's face, waiting first for the boom of the missile, then for the all-clear on the radio, with no one to talk to or be with in the long minutes in between. To avoid that situation, many singles moved in with parents and old friends; some, such as those employed in hospitals, slept at their workplaces; yet others teamed up with partners of convenience, old or new beaus. Dr. Ami Shaked, a sexologist, explained that the "need for togetherness makes singles less selective than in ordinary times" and that "physical contact is especially significant in times of tension and distress. . . . Walls come down and people are more open" (Shaked, 1991, p. 28).

Shaked warned, however, that "without some sort of common base, the relationship could end with a bang after the war." Similarly, moving back in with parents could also have its drawbacks, especially for people who had conflicted relationships with them to begin with. The journalist Aviva Kroll (1991) quotes a young man who tells that, back on his parents' turf during the war, all the old power struggles and the need to fight for his privacy and individuality started over again even though he thought he had resolved the problems years earlier. Bergman (1991) reports similar pressures on a 21-year-old patient of his when she went back to live with her mother and brother for the duration of the war. What we see in these examples, however, is that even where the relationship was problematic, people still preferred being with their families than by themselves during the war.

For noncustodial divorcees, mostly men, the hardships of aloneness could be compounded by the separation from their children. In many cases, the parent who had left the family home felt a strong desire to be with his children. The dilemma is treated in a collection of anecdotes, *Three in the Sealed Room*, by the journalists Amnon Dankner, Amnon Levy, and Ron Maiberg (1991). The anecdotes were originally published in an enormously popular newspaper column, and they spoofed the war and people's behavior in it. One of the stories goes as follows:

> I met an old friend who looked completely beat. "You can't image what a nightmare this is for me," he said. "My daughter from my previous marriage is on a kibbutz down South in the Northern Negev with my ex-wife; my son from my present marriage is with his mother up North in Afula. To see them I have to drive 600 kilometers a day. I'm exhausted. I'm living alone in our apartment that has an atomic bomb shelter and looks like a penthouse, and I'm dying to bring everyone home. . . . " "Nu," I asked him, "and why don't you?" "Because they're scared out of their wits in the city," he said. "The baby won't go into the Mamat (special gasproof tent for babies), my older daughter is hysterical, and besides I can't be with all of them at the same time. And on top of everything else, I can't stand my ex-wife's husband." (p. 100)

This spoof touches on several recurring problems of the war, including the search for security along with comfort, people's fears of being in the high-risk "city," and the difficulty of getting unwilling infants into their gasproof tents. Most tellingly, it deals with the dual problem of the divorced parent who remained out in the cold. As the narrator puts it, the divorced individual is torn between the strong desire to be with his former family, especially his children, and the great difficulty that entails, as people are kept apart both by geographic distance and by their inability to get along with each other.

## THE EXPLOSION AFTER

It is perhaps ironic that even though the family as a unit was more involved in the Gulf War than in any other war in Israel, few studies were carried out on it, and hard data from other sources are extremely limited. Two behavioral indicators that we thought might provide more concrete information about the pressure the Gulf War exerted on the family are divorce and family violence, but figures are hard to come by.

The data available are both provocative and highly imperfect. The picture seems to be that both divorce and family violence were put on hold for the duration of the war only to break out with the ceasefire in Iraq at the end of February and the lifting of the immediate threat to Israel.

According to a number of newspaper reports, divorce proceedings were put on hold, and fewer new petitions were filed (for example, Chen S., 1991). At the same time, new battles erupted over the children, among both divorced and married couples. Noncustodial divorced parents living abroad or outside the missile strike zones petitioned to have their children stay with them during the war. In united families where one parent, usually the mother, wanted to go abroad with the children, there were instances where the other parent obtained a court order to keep the children from leaving Israel. Unfortunately, the 1991 divorce figures are not yet available, so we have no way of knowing for certain the outcome of these and other war-engendered conflicts. Other wars in Israel, however, have been followed by an upsurge in divorce.

With regard to family violence, although there is little consensus as to its etiology, what we do know suggests that it should have increased during the Gulf War. It is generally agreed that frustration and family isolation—both of which were major occurrences in the Gulf War—increase the likelihood of family violence (Dollard, Doob, Mowrer, & Sears, 1939). Writing in Israel during the Gulf War, Ofra Ayalon (1991) predicted that the "no-exit situation" created by the forced intimacy and close confinement during the war could foster an increase in violence in families already prone to using violence to deal with their problems. Her contention was that with social contacts restricted and other outlets for aggression (that is, at work, on the road) blocked or greatly reduced by the war, the pent-up frustrations would be released within the family. At the same time, it can be argued that there are fewer deterrents to family violence during wartime than there ordinarily are. Gelles (1981, 1983, 1985) argues that the absence of effective social control of what goes on in the family lowers the price a family member has to pay for his violence and thereby increases the likelihood of its occurring. Even in peacetime, the authorities are loath to intervene in family quarrels and to punish or remove a violent member. They could be expected to have been even less zealous during wartime, and especially during the Gulf War, when they were busy with the danger to the population as a whole.

What actually happened during the war seems to have been more complex.

On the one hand, there seems to have been an increase in family friction expressed in verbal and low-grade physical abuse. This is suggested by the marked rise in complaints of physical and verbal abuse that were received during the first week or so of the war on a hotline run by Na'amat, a large Israeli women's organization, in Jerusalem. According to Tania Lif, who ran the hotline, there were many more calls describing abuse of children, spouses, and elderly parents. Lif says that the abuse seems to have been triggered by everyday conflicts, such as whether to seal the room, to wear or not wear the mask, or to stop up the crack under the door with a wet rag or not. She further relates that the "power struggles were now fought out over the sealed room, the children, and, in cases where the extended family came together, brothers, sisters, and in-laws too" (Gal N., 1991).

At the same time, more serious violence seems to have been curbed. Ronit Lev-Ari, a criminologist working for Na'amat, reported the same low-level conflict around gas masks, sealed rooms, and children but emphasized, "The first days of the war we didn't receive any complaints by battered wives. The general tension dwarfed the other tensions" (Shaked, 1991, p. 28). Even more tellingly, two of our students (Braker & Gilad, 1991) working in the emergency room of the Sheba Medical Center, one of the larger hospitals in the central area, reported that during the war only 5.7% of applications to the emergency room were for injuries caused by family violence, as opposed to the usual 60%. Unfortunately, it is difficult to know what portion of the difference is attributable to a decline in serious violence in the family and what portion to the increase in war-related emergencies, from problems breathing with the gas masks to the multitude of minor injuries incurred in the Scud attacks. Nonetheless, it does seem that, contrary to professional expectations, family violence did not increase with the stresses of the war, and even decreased. It may be that the life threat of the war made it necessary for violence-prone family members to develop alternative ways of dealing with their frustrations.

However, once the tension subsided, there seems to have been a renewed surge of violence. According to data supplied by Ronit Lev-Ari (1992) the last week of the war, battered wives again began to complain to the Na'amat hotline. Moreover, the rate of wife murder rose substantially. Forty-two women were killed by their husbands in 1991, the year of the Gulf War, as opposed to 18 in 1992.

Unfortunately, these figures are partial and difficult to interpret, since there are no large-scale empirical studies to provide a reliable picture. They do suggest, however, that even if most families coped adequately with the stresses of the war, in some the added strain seriously undermined the ability of the members to function as a family unit.

# 4

# Men and Women at War

## MEN AND WOMEN AT WAR: THE WARRIOR AND THE HOMEMAKER

Other than childbirth, little so clearly embodies the demarcation of male and female gender roles as warfare. Men go out and fight; women mind the house and kids. Men protect their wives and children; women wait for their husbands and sons to come back, and they welcome or mourn them at battle's end. Whether biological or social factors or both are responsible, the pattern remains, and whatever exceptions may be found only prove the rule.

It is thus not surprising that in time of war traditional gender roles are reinforced. Men are expected to be more "masculine," women more "feminine." This is no less true in Israel than anywhere else, even though women in this country serve in the military as both conscripts and career officers.

Ready illustration can be found in the 1973 Yom Kippur War. Analyzing the differences between men's and women's roles during that war, two prominent Israeli sociologists, Rivkah Bar-Yosef and Dorit Padan-Eisenstark (1977), point out that, as in all previous wars in Israel, traditional ascriptive sex roles reemerged and were strengthened, and their legitimacy was reinforced. As they describe it, the mobilization of the men divided the population into two distinct groups: active men and passive women and children.

They support their conclusion with a welter of descriptions and newspaper accounts, of which several are especially telling. Two days after the outbreak of the war, one article observes of Tel Aviv: "The streets, the cinemas, every place was suddenly so feminine. It's almost embarrassing for a man to make his way through the city. Why wasn't he called up? What is he still doing here?" (Why wasn't he, 1973). The assumption is not only that men should be away fighting and that only women stay home, but that fighting is "masculine" and staying at home is "feminine." Another journalist, quoting a soldier's sardonic comments shortly after the Israel Defense Forces (IDF) recaptured the West Bank of the Suez Canal, similarly points up the widespread assumption that the man's "place" is on the front and the woman's at home. As the soldier described it, "Africa," an area of Egypt conquered by the IDF, "became a closed men's club. We even placed MPs at the airports and on the bridges to remove anything that looked like a woman" (Avidar, 1973).

Since the soldier's job is valued more than the mother–homemaker's—if not at all times, then certainly during the war when the nation's security is at stake—the sharpening of the gender role dichotomy during wartime highlights the disparity between social reality and whatever ideals and aspirations for sexual equality that Israeli women hold. Yet another newspaper citation relates a woman's dissatisfaction with the disparity: "The war began and in one fell swoop our liberated woman's consciousness disappeared. Very quickly we were back in the days when the man went out to war to protect his tribe and the woman stayed home, and when he got back all she could do was to be gentle with him, take care of him, and trust in his ability to defend her from all evil" (Avidar, 1973).

If the gender polarization makes some sense in wars where there is active combat, it is hard to justify in a war where there is no active combat and men and women alike hurry to their sealed room or shelter and tape up the door. Nonetheless, even in the Gulf War, where whatever threat there was hovered equally over the sexes and there was no real division between protector and protected, men were still conceived of as the warriors, and women were seen as the weaker, less capable sex minding the home fires.

This dichotomy could be seen in all sorts of separate details that together formed a pattern. For example, one of the major decisions of the war, the closing and reopening of the schools, was made by 21 men, even though practically all of the teachers in Israel are women and the decision had far greater impact on the women and children who had to stay at home than on the men who could go on with their lives in any case. To be sure, this distortion was a carryover of inequalities inherent in the system and merely pointed up the questionable propriety of men

managing a school system where the overwhelming majority of employees are women.

More glaring was the outright sexual discrimination in the radio
broadcasting system. As noted in Chapter 1, Israel's three government
radio stations merged during the war. In the temporary personnel cut-
back that followed, all the female announcers were sent home, and only
the men were left to broadcast the news, moderate the discussions, and
play the cassettes or records. Why that was done is difficult to fathom on
purely practical grounds. The broadcasts came from Jerusalem, which
was not targeted during the war, and the work entailed no particular
danger or physical effort. The explanation that offers itself is the deep-
rooted assumption that war is men's business, not women's.

Indeed, this assumption seems to have pervaded the entire wartime
economy. In previous wars, women filled in the factories and offices for
the men away at the front. In the Gulf War, with no front, men went out
to work—to keep the hobbling wartime economy going—while many
women who ordinarily worked were forced to stay home to mind the
children because no alternative arrangements were made. More will be
said of this below.

Here the point I wish to make is that as far as gender roles were
concerned, the Gulf War entailed two contradictory aspects. One is that,
in contrast to other wars, men and women were subjected to the same
life threat. Gone was the difference between the man risking his life on
the front and the woman staying safe at home. The Scuds aimed at the
civilian population threatened men and women equally.

The other contradictory aspect is that the traditional wartime
gender-role polarizations nonetheless occurred, often in practice and
even more essentially in the mind-set behind the practice. This means
that while men and women experienced the same stressor on the macro
level of life threat, their day-to-day experiences and stresses were different. The remainder of this chapter will focus on these two aspects of the
war. First it will discuss in greater detail the specific stresses that the war
created for men and women. Then it will look at a range of studies of
their reactions and responses to the war.

## IDENTITY UNDERMINED: WHAT IS A MAN?

If war is generally considered men's business, in Israel male identity
is perhaps more closely bound up with the warrior role than it is in other
societies. The link has several sources. The first, as always, is myth: the

myth is the contrast between the weak and persecuted Diaspora Jew who did not have the wherewithal or will to defend himself or his family, and the "new Jew," the strong, powerful Israeli who, for the better part of the century, has been warding off one or another enemy who would destroy him and his country.

In the reality of Israeli men, and women too, myth joins with history. In actuality, most Israeli men spend a good part of their lives in the military, in active reserves, and in the periodic wars and flare-ups in which this country has been involved. Indeed, a large number of Israeli men have fought in two and even three or more wars or smaller-scale "operations." Since Israel is under constant threat, the vital role of the military in the survival of the country and of the people in it adds untold importance to the warrior role.

During the Gulf War, the Israeli man in the prime of life was spared the major and massive stress of combat: the close threat of injury and death. The life danger was further off; he was not immersed in views of mangled corpses, and he did not have to endure the physical hardships of the battlefield or the separation from his family at home. On the other hand, though, he was deprived of weapons with which to defend himself and his family, and deprived too of the ability to act, which gives one a feeling of control, even if illusory, and serves as an avenue for the release of fear, aggression, and frustration. The forced passivity, as difficult as it may have been for women, was probably much more so for men; for, as we know from the literature, while women generally cope with stress by turning inward, men tend to cope by taking action (Barnett, Biener, & Baruch, 1987). Moreover, to add insult to injury, it was not only that men were booted out of their traditional "place" in the defense of the country and deprived of their preferred coping mechanism, but they also were planted, of all places, at home with their wives and children, which is not their natural domain at any time, and especially not during war.

The policy of restraint in the Gulf War, which kept men at home with the traditionally helpless and weak women and children, thus undermined one of the major pillars of the identity of the Israeli man; placed him in an embarrassing, somewhat humiliating position; and threatened his masculinity. This is suggested, among other things, by the humor that the situation provoked. A satirical television program that became popular during the war had a very small man facing his very large wife, and he was so scared that he kept injecting himself with the nerve-gas antidote provided with the gas masks. The skit illustrates the feeling of role reversal and diminution of the Israeli male that the policy evidently created. Another joke making the rounds during the war was

"I don't need a wet rag to stop up the threshold of the sealed room because I have my husband." The term "wet rag" denotes a special floor-cleaning cloth used in Israel, and in conversation is used to refer to a man one can "wipe the floor with," so to speak. Like the television skit, this joke hinges on the diminution of the Israeli man during the war and conveys the message that he was somehow in the wrong place at the wrong time. The frightened little men of these barbed depictions were not doing their job, not fulfilling their male responsibility, and not fighting for their families; consequently, they were worthless.

Whether this perception was held primarily by the men, by the women, or by both is impossible to ascertain. Nor is it certain that all or even the majority of Israelis, of either sex, saw the matter in this way. The country's many new and not-so-new immigrants, from Ethiopia, Russia, Europe, and the Americas, may not have. Nonetheless, the sense of masculine debasement associated with the imposed inactivity during the Gulf war is a natural product of the typical Israeli upbringing and social climate of the last few generations, and it is unlikely that most of the men of those times escaped it.

Ironically, however, this ignoble ouster from the warrior role seems to have resulted in a denial of the threat on the part of men, which thrust women into the role of defender. In home after home, it was the woman who cross-taped the windows, sealed the rooms, bought the emergency provisions, and generally prepared the house for the upcoming war, while the men looked on with a skeptical and superior manner, denying that anything serious would happen. A satiric portrait drawn by the journalist Nira Russo (1991) depicts the situation:

If someone had observed us [her husband and herself] during the fearful and terrible week before the war, it would not have occurred to them that we had any relationship whatsoever. Every tension-filled thing I did to protect those near and dear to me, he saw as mad panic. After all, there are newspapers, commentators, the army, predictions. . . . The likelihood [of anything happening] is low. For the next few days till the end of the ultimatum we ran through a fixed script, which went like this: In the morning the woman (I) listened to the news, her face taut, with black bags under her eyes. As soon as it was over, she swung into action, frantically getting the house ready: sealing, mineral water, sheltering, defense, and preparedness. He, in contrast, took it easy. First he would switch the radio from the daily news magazine to a popular music station, for why confuse him with facts? Then it was time for his cigar and coffee at leisure in the garden. He looked on his wife's mad, unphotogenic runnings about with pitying ridicule. The message he conveyed, as always, was that another man, less tolerant and easy going, would already have given her a sever dressing down for this uncontrolled hysteria. What should we say—she's lucky. Being a broad-minded chap, he allows her to express her needs as the narrow-minded mother hen living with him who insists on spreading a blanket of protection over the house. All this, as long as she doesn't bother him too much. . . .

. . . As long as he's not forced to sleep in a sealed room (which, as everyone knows, is not good for your health) only because an unbalanced female decided that the Iraqis would keep their promise. From a forgiving pity he goes to pointed revenge: "I don't understand. You also read newspapers, and they all say that nothing will happen, and anything that does will be negligible."

The issue that Russo points to is not simply that men left the work for the women and became angry when they were pressed to participate. That could be attributed to the traditional division of labor that still pertains in most households, with women doing the jobs in and related to the home, and men doing the jobs outside. The issue in her eyes, and mine, is the blanket denial of the threat. It is not simply that her husband and other men she knew did not do their share in preparing for the war. It was that, along with the entire male establishment from the government through the media, they refused to take Saddam Hussein's threats seriously, insisting variously that he would not carry them out, that if he tried to he would not succeed, or that if he did manage to strike, any damage would be negligible. This denial lies behind the refusal of the men to take any action that could be seen as an acknowledgment of the threat and accounts for their supercilious contempt for the "hysterical females" who did acknowledge it.

Russo notes that the "complete detachment" that characterized the men before the war ended with the first missile strike. In my own experience, it persisted throughout the war, with my husband, to cite only one example, going through the emergency procedures only to placate the children and myself, or acting as if that were his only motive. The reasons that Russo suggests for this attitude are relevant to the matter of the threat to male identity. "You have to understand them," she quotes her forgiving women friends as saying. "After all, they're men."

This is the first time they're not actually in the army. They don't have the chance to shed blood for their country, and they themselves admit that the home front is many times as stressful. You know, after all, that in the army, they're with the guys, in action. And here they're suddenly stuck with the kids, and we have to understand how hard it is for them.

The sarcasm of the explanation notwithstanding, it points to the widespread awareness among women that their men were out of their element in the Gulf War, discomforted by not being able to "shed blood for their country" and stressed on the home front, where they were "suddenly stuck with the kids."

I believe that there was another element in the denial as well. It was difficult for men who were accustomed to being soldiers to conceive of a war, or of any real danger, in which they were not called up. In rather circular fashion, the reasoning, I believe, was, "since we're not being called up, nothing will happen (or, once the missiles started to fall, they reasoned that "nothing serious is happening"). The converse of this logic was, if something does, or did, happen, and we're not called up, what kind of men are we? The denial of the Iraqi danger thus served to sustain the sense of male identity that was under threat on the home front.

### ROLE CONFLICT

For women, the major stress was not so much the war's challenge to identity as role strain—the demand that women do two jobs at once, childcare and their paid work, and quite literally be in two places at the same time. The war greatly exacerbated a fundamental and trying conflict of working women in our time.

In comparison to the United States, Israel has fairly good childcare facilities. There are daycare centers open from seven to four o'clock, after-school programs that provide supervision for young children until three o'clock, and a rich network of private childcare workers for those who have the money to employ them. On the whole, however, these arrangements best serve women in part-time or government jobs with relatively short working hours and are inadequate for women with more demanding positions.

During the war, even these arrangements were greatly reduced. For the first three weeks, schools and daycare facilities were closed. When they were reopened, parents had to do school duty to help the teachers in case of an air raid. This meant that one of the adults in the family, usually the mother, had to spend about 1 workday in 8 or 10 days at school for each child. Most after-school facilities remained shut, and many private arrangements fell apart. Some women found that their babysitters had joined the exodus from the high-risk areas. Grandparents, who in peacetime might come to the rescue in an emergency, were wary of taking on the responsibility, fearing that they might not be quick or dexterous enough to cope in case of an alarm. Babies and toddlers were particularly difficult to find alternative care for. To go outside with them, one had to carry on one's back their bulky gasproof baby tent. Not everyone was prepared to do that. Nor was everyone prepared to shove a screaming and kicking baby into the tent in case of an alarm. Moreover, as already noted, children who could ordinarily be left alone or in the care of older siblings for short periods could not be left on their own during the war.

Many large firms and institutions soon realized that if they wanted to stay in operation they would have to provide temporary childcare facilities. But small employers generally could not, and many working mothers fell outside the net. They were expected to be at work but could not find arrangements for their children. This created particular dilemmas and hardships for women. All women who stayed home lost pay. Single and divorced mothers were especially hard hit. They generally had a smaller social network from which to enlist assistance, so had a harder time getting to work. At the same time, the income they lost by staying home was usually not the family's second income, but its first and only income. Women in the helping professions were torn between caring for their own children and providing important and sometimes vital services for their clients.

Women who found childcare arrangements—a competent babysitter or member of the extended family willing to fill in for them—or who shared childcare with their husbands did not necessarily have peace of mind. With the ever-present danger of the Scuds, having one's children in someone else's care was decidedly a worry, especially in the high-risk Tel Aviv and Haifa areas. Working mothers are often split between the demands of work and home. During the Gulf War, that split was greatly exacerbated. I think it is safe to say that many women who did show up at their places of work were there mainly in body, with their spirits at home with their kids. This is not to say that men were not worried or concerned. They were. But since childcare is still considered—by men and women alike—mainly the responsibility of women, with the men playing only (ever-larger) secondary roles, it was the women who bore the brunt of the worry and guilt about their children when they were away at work.

To illustrate the role strain, I draw on the example of women career officers in the Mental Health Department of the IDF Medical Corps. The example is handy because I am personally familiar with it, and also because it contains in a nutshell what I see as the dilemma of the working woman in general and during the Gulf War in particular.

The IDF is a large organization run by men but with a substantial female work force. In some divisions, the Medial Corps among them, women hold responsible posts and play an important role. In the Department of Mental Health, which consists primarily of career officers, there is an almost equal number of men and women. Since the IDF is a largely civilian army with a relatively small career core, during most wars large numbers of reservists are called up, to the Mental Health Department no less than to other corps. The large-scale call-ups change the proportion of men and women in the department, and the situation necessitates changes in how the sexes are deployed. Most of the men, both reservists and career officers, are sent to the medical and mental health stations on or near the front, while the women remain in their departmental posts or are assigned to hospitals and other treatment facilities within Israel, from where they go back home for the night. This was the pattern in all of Israel's wars prior to the Gulf War. During the Gulf War there was no mass call-up of reserves, so the gender distribution remained as it was in peacetime and, for the most part, both men and women continued at the tasks they had done previously, and both went home at night. At most, people of both sexes were called on to work late. Nonetheless, the female workers were under considerable role pressure.

A case in point is that of Major Mimi Samovski, a mental health officer posted at one of the IDF's largest bases. Both her work and home were in Tel Aviv. She and her husband, also a career officer, a lieutenant colonel, had a one-year-old baby. The couple's babysitter was among those who fled the country before the January 15 deadline. The Samonskis had no relatives in Tel Aviv or anyone else to replace the babysitter. Inevitably, one of the parents would have to stay with the baby, and there was no question which one it would be. Both agreed that Lieutenant Colonel Samovski's work was more important and demanded all his time. Major Samovski was torn. The army needed her but her baby needed her more. She took her daughter, and they waited out the war with Grandma in Beer Sheva in the south of the country.

The inner conflict that this engendered was so intense that in an interview a full two years after the war, Major Samovski still spoke of it with strong emotion. She told that she had felt as if she were being torn by two horses pulling in opposite directions. "I never knew the meaning of conflict till then," she said. "All the while I was in Beer Sheva, I felt guilty that I wasn't doing what I was supposed to be. At the beginning, a lot of people pressured me to come back. Then they began spreading stories that I was shirking my responsibility, that I'd run away, that I'd abandoned my clients."

Yet another example is the situation faced by the head of the Women's Army Corps, Brigadier General Hedva Almog. The IDF's only (and token) woman brigadier general, Almog told of her dilemma in an interview with the IDF weekly *BaMahane* (Peleg, 1991). Brigadier General Almog's situation was different from Major Samovski's. Her home was about as close as you could get to a "liberated" household. For years, while she pursued her career in the military, her husband was the one to make the concessions. When the war broke out, no one in the family saw any reason to change the pattern. Mother went to her work in the army in Tel Aviv, and she stayed overnight when she had to. Father remained in Haifa with the kids; if he had to make adjustments in his work, he would, as he always had, even though his job at the Haifa port was also considered high priority in wartime.

Then came the Scud attacks. One night Brigadier General Almog was in Tel Aviv, when missiles landed almost simultaneously in the two cities. Her husband and children were on their own in Haifa in the midst of a missile attack. From that evening on, she told the reporter, she decided she would return to Haifa when she finished work, no matter what the hour, so that she could spend the night with her family. To cap matters, the following week her husband was called up for civil defense duty, which could not be deferred. Other childcare arrangements had to be made, and the overnight stays at work had to end, whether she wanted them to or not.

This example shows that even a liberated woman with a fully cooperative husband in a liberated household encountered role problems during the war. The problems stemmed both from her emotions, from the typically feminine feeling that she could not leave her family to face the threat on their own, and from the social and military norms that make it impossible to defer a man's civil defense call-up, even if his wife is a brigadier general.

The conflict derives ultimately from the equation between soldier and man. It is clear that a soldier's first duty is to the army, and that in time of war the army takes precedence over his family. Thus it is difficult for me even to conceive of a male brigadier general, or a lower-ranking male career officer for that matter, rushing home from his post because his wife and children might have needed him, as Brigadier General Almog did. To be sure, there were conscripts and reservists who asked to be released from duty on account of family problems. But a male career officer who decided to go home to spend the night with his wife and children in the middle of a national emergency, or even a much lesser crisis, would have been laughed out of the army. It is unlikely he would even have thought of doing so. But for Brigadier General Almog and women throughout the army services, the issue was much more complicated. They were both soldiers and women, and their first duty was not nearly as clearly defined. The conflict arose for women because army and family were both first—or, to put it more precisely, family was first but army was only a hair's breath away.

These examples, as different as they are, show that the care of house and child usually devolves to women, and all the more so in wartime. The dilemma is not an easy one to solve. During wartime, when resources are pulled taut, finding solutions may be even harder. Going back to our two examples, finding ad hoc childcare for very small children may have been close to a "mission impossible," and no social setup can do anything to alleviate the guilt and anxiety a woman may feel about leaving her family to fend for themselves. If these particular situations are indicative, the problem has two dimensions: one social, one emotional. It may be that neither is entirely soluble. The emotional difficulty is almost certainly not. The social problem, inadequate childcare, may be amenable to only a partial solution.

The IDF addressed neither issue. In this, it fell behind other large institutions in Israel, from the country's public universities through scores of private companies. Nor, in my opinion, is the reason simply that the matter is outside the army's domain. The Israeli army is, and always has been involved in a wide range of social issues, from immigrant absorption through education. Rather, the core of the problem seems to be the adherence to gender-role typing in an institution that, when all is said and done, sees itself as an expression of maleness.

Something of this can be seen in the following letter by Major Eitan Abraham, who is in charge of Mental Health Center Command, to the chief of IDF Mental Health Services. The letter questions the ability of women to fill important army positions in view of the difficulties encountered in the Gulf War. It voices two concerns: that women who could not find childcare arrangements did not show up for work and that women could not perform in the army's "emergency routine," which requires all soldiers to be on call around the clock:

re: functioning of mothers in the Mental Health Department during emergencies.
1. The missile bombardment on the civilian population and the resulting "emergency routine" has put into question the ability of mothers to fill vital positions in the army.
2. In the Central Command Headquarters there are 11 married mental health workers of whom 6 are mothers. A number of problems arose in the group:
   a. The commander of the infirmary did not find an arrangement for her daughter and left for Beer Sheva without giving notice.
   b. One of the mental health officers did everything in her power to avoid night duty.
   c. Another officer who had just returned from maternity leave gave a number of personal reasons—husband fired, mother-in-law in hospital, problematic financial situation—that made her unable to participate in the emergency routine.
   d. There are two other similar cases that indicate that this is not an isolated situation.
3. Similarly, a number of female mental health officers have advised me that they will not be able to answer to any call-up.

4. I must report that a number of mothers did manage to solve this conflict and report for duty as needed.

5. This has caused dissatisfaction among those officers who are on duty all the time and has also undermined the credibility of our services in time of need.

6. Work conditions in the IDF take into account the needs of mothers, but in an emergency all military personnel must be available at all times. . . .

7. I do not want to generalize to all women serving in the military, but I think the time has come to redefine their duties with the head of the Women's Corps.

8. These expectations must be clear when they take on military employment, and sanctions must be clear for all who are incapable of fulfilling them.

While there is no arguing with the major's contention that women in responsible positions should be expected to be there no less than men, the letter totally ignores the genuine dilemma of women expected to be in two places at once and suggests no means of resolving or even alleviating the problem. Childcare is not mentioned once. Without suggesting any alternative, the only "solution" the writer offers is to penalize women for nonperformance. There is also the suggestion, more hinted at than offered outright, that he would like to see the army revert to old gender divisions, with the men in responsible positions and the women kept down in the ranks.

To reiterate, the picture we have is of men and women facing the same life threat on the macro level, but each having to contend with their own specific gender-related stresses on the micro level. The shared life threat made it seem possible and potentially informative to study the responses of men and women comparatively—to ask questions like, Did they respond similarly or differently to the war? If differently, how?

## FINDINGS OF GENDER DIFFERENCES

Numerous empirical studies were carried out bearing on these questions. In most of them, the gender comparison was only one among several issues. The studies all point to similar gender differences. Women endorsed greater fear and poorer coping than men.

The telephone survey by Lavie et al. (1991) of wartime sleep disturbances (discussed in Chapter 2) among a random sample of 100 men and 100 women from all over Israel found that although a similar proportion of men and women reported difficulty in falling asleep and waking up in midsleep, significantly more women than men reported having both problems (21% versus 4.1%). Moreover, of the six people (3% of the sample) who admitted to using sleeping pills, five were women. The authors note that these findings are in keeping with reports by both American and Israeli researchers of a similar preponderance of complaints of insomnia among women and much higher sleeping-pill use by women than men.

Gal (1992), in his study of four groups of adults residing in three different parts of the country (discussed in Chapter 2), found that women reported being more fearful than men. A considerably higher percentage of women than men described the war as either "deathly frightening" or "very frightening" (28.4% versus 8.4%). Women assessed their level of fear on the day after the first missile attack as significantly higher than men (averaging 5.1 on a 7-point scale as opposed to 4.2 among the men), though there were no gender differences in the fear levels reported after the two subsequent missile attacks.

The IDF Department of Behavior Sciences' (DBS) study of the general population (described in Chapter 2) provides a broader, but similar, picture of gender differences in response to the war. Differences were found in men's and women's assessments of their functioning and coping, in one aspect of their actual functioning, and in their somatic complaints.

In the area of functioning, men had a higher opinion of their conduct in the war than women did of their own. More specifically, men consistently reported higher levels of familiarity with the protective devices than women, viewed themselves as more knowledgeable about what to do in case of an attack, saw themselves as better able to help their children put on their gas masks, and reported less need for additional information about the protective devices and procedures.

Men also saw themselves as coping better with the war than women saw themselves. In each of the six separate assessments of coping made between January 30 and February 24, a higher proportion of men than women rated their coping as good or very good (the top two grades on a 4-point scale). The gender difference was initially about 20%, then decreased to 9% by the end of the war, showing increasing habituation on the part of women.

In the realm of action, men seem to have adhered somewhat less to the emergency instructions than women. Although the same proportion of men and women took shelter at the sound of the alarm, put on their masks, and took their protective kits along when they left the house, throughout most of the war significantly more men than women removed their gas masks before the order to do so was given. The gap closed only in the last week of the war, when compliance with the emergency instructions went down throughout the population.

Also on the level of functioning, men reported less disruption in their daily routine than women. In an assessment taken toward the end of the war (February 24–25, 1991), 37% of the women surveyed reported that the war disrupted their daily routine to a high degree, as opposed to only 22% of the men.

With regard to symptoms, women also reported more somatic complaints in the sealed room than men: more burning sensations, tears, breathing difficulties, and excessive perspiration. Throughout most of the war, the difference was about two to one, with twice as many women as men reporting symptoms; during the first survey on January 18, it was almost three to one.

The findings all seem to point to men's greater sense of mastery during the war. This would be consistent with the point made above that war belongs to the masculine domain. In the view of the DBS, it is only logical that men would feel more self-confident, in greater control, and less afraid than women in a war situation, for which they have had preparation and practice. On the other hand, the finding that a greater proportion of women than men reported that the war substantially disrupted their daily routine seems to reflect different gender experiences: while men continued to go to work, at most coming home early, women's schedules—whether inside or outside the house—were radically upset by the added burden of childcare during the war. The finding that women felt they coped less well during the war could reflect the objective fact that they had more to cope with than men did.

Two studies attempted to assess men's and women's responses to the war by comparing wartime with non-wartime measures of emotions. They too found gender differences.

One was the study by Ben-Zur and Zeidner (1991), discussed in Chapter 2, which compared a "crisis group" of 500 subjects (39% men, 61% women) assessed during the war with a "norm" group with a similar proportion of males and females assessed a few years earlier. This study found that the women in both groups registered significantly higher anxiety than the men and, moreover, that their anxiety went up more than the men's from prewar levels. Findings showed that the war accounted for 29% of the total variance in the women's anxiety scores as opposed to only 13% of the variance in the men's scores.

The authors also found that during the war, women reported higher levels of tension, fear, and depression than men (on one-item rating scales) and a higher frequency of somatic symptoms. More women reported loss of appetite or overeating (72% of women versus 46% of men); fatigue (71% versus 58%); insomnia (70% versus 44%); headaches (45% versus 25%); backache or neck ache (42% versus 18%); breathing difficulties (37% versus 17%); and constipation or diarrhea (34% versus 9%).

The authors offer two explanations for these differences: that women tend to respond more emotionally to crises than men and that the experience Israeli men have with military events made them better able to deal with the stress of war than their less-experienced female counterparts.

The other study, carried out by Lomranz and Eyal (1994) of Tel Aviv University, was a longitudinal investigation of changes in depressive mood in reaction to the war. This study queried 3,204 subjects, 57.5% of them women and 42.5% men, representative of Israel's over-18 Jewish population, excluding kibbutznikim. The subjects were tested in four waves: before the threat of war (June 1990), under the treat of war (December 1990), during the war (February 1991), and soon after the war ended (March 1991). In each wave different subjects filled out Lubin's Depression Adjective Checklist (Lubin, 1967).

The study found that men and women were substantially similar in depressive mood both before and after the war, but differed significantly during the war. To begin with, in December, under the threat of war, the depressive mood of both genders rose in virtually equal measure from its June level (though the difference did not reach significance). During the war, however, the level of the women's depressive mood shot up significantly, while the men's remained almost exactly as it had been. In March, with the war's end, the depressive mood of both genders went back down to its June level.

The findings parallel Ben-Zur and Zeidner's (1991) findings on anxiety and are consistent with the other studies showing that women had stronger emotional reactions to the war than men. Unlike the other authors, however, Lomranz and Eyal do not take their findings at face value. They attribute the stability in the men's depressive mood to denial, which, in their view, is the typical way that Israeli men cope with threats on which they are powerless to act. They attribute the intensification of depressive mood among women to the heavy emotional burden that women bore during the war: women, they point out, bore the weight of the responsibility of their children under extremely uncertain circumstances; fought a double battle against the men's denial, on the one hand, and the potential dangers of the war, on the other; and played not only the traditional female role of family caregiver, but also the classic male role of defender and protector, as they readied their homes for the war. The authors suggest that these double, and sometimes conflicting, roles created a heavy emotional burden that expressed itself in depressive mood.

The studies discussed above focused largely on emotional and cognitive responses to the war. Shapira, Marganitt, Roziner, Shochet, Bar, and Shemer's (1991) wide-ranging survey of the employees of 10 hospitals in various parts of Israel examined behavioral intentions. The survey was taken to provide information on the extent to which hospitals would be able to rely on personnel reporting to work under the risk of toxic exposure in the aftermath of an unconventional attack—a risk that all family members would face if one of them left the sealed room before the all-clear. To this end, the authors sent out an anonymous questionnaire, which asked the employees whether they would be willing to report for emergency duties immediately after a chemical attack should they be summoned to do so. The findings from the 1374 responses show that a significantly higher proportion of males (61%) than females (34%) said they would be willing to report.

The authors' analyses suggest that both different anxiety levels and the role perception of mothers as being primarily responsible for the family's children play a part in the difference. On the one hand, the greater projected willingness of men to report was consistent across all study categories—whatever the family size, the age of the youngest child residing in the household, the respondent's specific profession, and the role of the respondent in the hospital's disaster plan. Moreover, women with no children showed significantly less willingness to report to work (40%) than men with no children (63%). These findings suggest that gender differences in anxiety were behind the figures.

On the other hand, a significantly smaller percentage of mothers with children living at home (32%) than women with no children (40%) indicated willingness to report. Furthermore, mothers with two or three children were significantly less willing to report (28–29%) than mothers of one child (40%), while fathers' willingness to return to work increased (though nonsignificantly) with family size. These findings emphasize the part played by the mother role.

## METHODOLOGICAL ARTIFACT, ACKNOWLEDGMENT OF DISTRESS, OR REAL GENDER DIFFERENCE?

Observations of emotional responses of men and women in the Gulf War are consistent with many previous studies that found that women are more likely than men to report symptoms of anxiety and depression (for example, Murphy, Sobol, Neff, Olivier, & Leighton, 1984; Weissman & Kelerman, 1977). Women have repeatedly been shown to be more likely than men to manifest psychological distress in the face of adversity, whether from stressful life events or from catastrophic events such as natural disasters or war (Strumpfer, 1970). Despite this consistency, however, the findings in the Gulf War studies reported above are open to interpretation. Some differences in interpretation have already been recorded above. Here I suggest several ways of looking at the results.

First, it is possible that the findings are a methodological artifact derived from biased selection of outcome measures. To begin with, all of the measures are self-reports, none of them physiological. However, it has been shown that women report more distress than men even when their physiological responses are the same as or milder than men's. Collins (1985) shows that although females are *less* prone than males to react with an increase in circulating epinephrine (or adrenalin) when experiencing mental stressors, their self-reports of subjective discomfort and lack of confidence are *greater* than those of males. Similarly, Everly and Humphry (1980) have pointed out that women tend more than men to *interpret* their levels of physiological arousal as reflecting negative affect.

In a similar vein, the outcome measures tapped mainly the inhibitive behaviors—fear, anxiety, depression, and worry—that are characteristic of women under stress, rather than the proactive behaviors, such as aggression and substance abuse, typical of men (Everly, 1989; Gibbs, 1989; Gleser, Green, & Winget, 1981; Newman, 1989). Indeed there is a substantial body of disaster research (Gibbs, 1989) showing differential gender manifestations of distress precisely along these lines. Female survivors of traumas have been found to show more anxiety somatic complaints, or social withdrawal, whereas male survivors exhibit more alcohol abuse and belligerence (Gleser et al., 1981; Janoff-Bullman & Frieze, 1987). Other studies have found that while women showed more depression, somatization, or psychiatric symptomatology, men showed more physical illness (Bennet, 1970; Cowan & Murphy, 1985).

A second interpretation of the findings is that they are an outcome of women's greater readiness to *acknowledge* and report their distress. This interpretation is consistent with Lomranz and Eyal's view, cited above, that the stability they found in men's depressive mood during the war reflected denial, or disinclination to disclose distress. This interpretation is also consistent with the satiric picture of masculine denial drawn by Russo (1991). It is certainly commonplace that differential social expectations, not only in Israel but worldwide, permit women to express weakness but forbid or discourage that admission in men. In the words of Nasjleti (1980, p. 271), "From early childhood boys learn that masculinity means not depending on anyone, not being weak, not being passive, not being a loser in confrontation, in short, not being a victim." The view that the findings reflect these differential expectations is supported by studies showing that women adopt the sick role and seek care more easily than men (for example, Woods & Hulka, 1979).

During the Gulf War, which posed a challenge to the Israeli man's sense of masculinity, the pressure to maintain a facade of strength and self-assurance may have been all the stronger. In this interpretation, the men's self-reported self-confidence about the emergency procedures, their sense of coping well, their readiness to remove their gas masks before instructed to, and their comparatively lower endorsement of anxiety, depression, sleep disturbances, and somatic symptoms can all reflect the need to protect the masculinity that was challenged by this war that was not a war. While it may well be that men, many of whom had experienced the more immediately horrific and threatening dangers of combat, were truly less frightened than women by the threat of the Gulf War, it would certainly have been more embarrassing for men who were frightened to admit it, even to themselves, and more threatening to their self-esteem.

The third interpretation is that women did in fact experience higher levels of distress than men during the Gulf War. The difference could be rooted in one or more of several factors, ranging from different male and female coping styles, to the role conflict faced by women and the different sensitivities of the two sexes.

## Coping Style

The findings could be accounted for by the possibility that the coping strategies women employ dispose them to higher levels of distress. Pearlin and Schooler (1978) argue that the coping strategies women employ are less effective in buffering the psychological effects of life stress than the strategies men use. Others contend that women's socialization produces susceptibility to stress through the learning of helplessness (for example, Randolph & Rahe, 1979). This line of argument views women's coping style as less functional than men's. However, the evidence, with regard both to the gender differentiation of coping styles and to the effectiveness of these styles, is far from conclusive.

## Role Conflict

For working women, the life-threat pressures of the Gulf War were compounded by the pressures of role strain. Gove (1972, 1979) and Gove and Tudor (1973) have observed that even under ordinary circumstances, more family role demands are made on women than on men and that the role of wife and mother is more likely to conflict with other role demands than that of husband and father. During the Gulf War, as we recall, the conflicts were intensified as schools, kindergartens, and childcare facilities were shut or curtailed, yet places of work reopened after a few days and adults were required to return. In many two-paycheck families, this meant that the husband returned to work without much ado, while the wife had to choose: either she remained at home, AWOL, to mind the children, or she went to work and left the children in someone else's care in a potentially dangerous situation. In either case, she could feel that she was neglecting an important responsibility.

## Different Sensitivities

The major source of stress in the Gulf War was the threat to one's own and others' lives and safety. The greater distress of women during the war may have derived from their tendency to be more sensitive to and involved with the needs and feelings of others than were men. It has been found, for example, that while men tend to be upset by work-related strains, women are more upset by interpersonal problems (Pearlin, 1975). It has been suggested that women are socialized to feel greater concern for their loved ones than men (Gilligan, 1982) and tend to be more affected than men by things that happen to people around them (Strobe & Strobe, 1983). Dohrenwend and Dohrenwend (1976) found, for instance, that when men and women were asked to list recent stressful incidents that had happened to them and to significant others, women reported a higher proportion of things that had happened to others than to themselves.

Not only the depth but also the extent of women's concern for others may be greater than men's. Women tend to cast a wider net into the social arena than men and to define more people as important to them (Barnett et al., 1987). It has been suggested that women's social involvement may predispose them to a "contagion of stress that is felt when adversity afflicts those to whom they are emotionally close." Kessler and Maleod (1984) argue that this sensitivity to the troubles of others accounts for women's greater vulnerability to stressful life events.

In the Gulf War, women's more acute sensitivities would have predisposed them to worry more than men about the many people around them who were under threat: their children, their parents, and near and distant family members and friends. Men may have been better able to distance themselves from other people's anxieties and to avoid the personal distress that women experienced from network events.

These interpretations need not be mutually exclusive. On the one hand, we have indirect evidence that men did feel distress during the Gulf War. One possible indication, discussed in the previous chapter, is the upsurge of family violence, including wife murder, that occurred in the aftermath of the war. Another indication was suggested in conversation by Ami Shaked, the director of sex therapy clinic at a major hospital in the Tel Aviv area, who reported an apparent increase in sexual problems among men. According to Shaked, shortly after the war men came to the clinic in increased numbers with sexual problems whose onset they located in or attributed to the war. At the same time, it is difficult to imagine that the intense role strain to which women were subjected and their heightened sensitivities to others would not have taken an emotional toll.

# 5

# Children in the Line of Fire

## CHILDREN AND ADULTS: SHARED EXPERIENCES, DIFFERENT EXPERIENCES

Children and adults shared the essential experience of the Gulf War— the threat of attack—to an extent to which they had rarely, if ever, shared war experiences in Israel before. In previous wars, with the exception of the 1948 War of Independence, the army had quickly moved the fighting beyond the country's borders, and the major threat to children was that their fathers and older brothers could be wounded or killed on the front. This threat was horrible, but, except for a few isolated air raids, children themselves were not targets and were relatively safe, along with their mothers and most other members of the household. In the Gulf War they were no safer than anyone else, and all but the youngest knew it.

The threat was brought home to children, as to adults, by the multitude of protective measures and the restrictions of the emergency routine. Like others in their homes, children were awakened by the sirens at night, hurried into the sealed room or shelter, and wore (or refused to wear) their gas masks while they waited for the all-clear. Some slept in their parents' bedroom, which had been turned into the sealed room; many slept in jogging suits so as to be in street clothes in case of an attack. Their meals and baths were moved up so as to be out of the way before the Scuds arrived. Many children were actively involved in sealing windows, taping up the doors of the sealed room, helping younger siblings or their parents on with their gas masks, or looking after elderly relatives (Mendler, 1991). Like their parents, too, children were exposed

to the deluge of war-related programming that began in the days before
the Coalition ultimatum expired, so they were able to grasp the menace
and realize that their lives were in danger. In short, this was a war whose
threat children could experience directly. As the journalist Ariella
Ringel-Hoffman (1991) describes it, this was "a filmed, mass mediaed,
talked about war [in which] children see everything, hear everything,
know everything" (pp. 4–5).

At the same time, children had to contend with particular pressures
of their own. In some ways, the war had more of an impact on the course
of children's lives than on the lives of adults. After the first four days,
when shops, schools, and offices were closed and parents and children
waited out the time together at home, adults returned to work, but
children did not return to school.

What lay behind the decision to keep the schools closed is beyond
the scope of this discussion. Consideration of the children's safety was
probably among the motives, along with uncertainties as to how long the
war would last and how damaging Iraq's expected attacks against Israel
would be. The immediate result of the decision, however, was that
school-age children were removed from their natural habitat in a time of
crisis. The closure of the schools for the first three weeks of the war
deprived children of the social support of their peers, the reassurance of
their teachers, and the steadying influence of familiar structures and
routines at precisely the time when they most needed them. The Ministry of Education, which was behind the decision to keep the schools
closed, was evidently aware of the hardship this entailed and, to mitigate
it, organized telephone hotlines that children and their parents could
call for advice and reassurance.

The return to work of the adult population compounded the dislocation inherent in the school closure. In a country with a high percentage of women in the labor force, the return to work gave rise to a variety
of scenarios, none of them conducive to children's peace of mind. In
some families the mother simply stayed home, or the mother and father
took turns minding the children. In others, children were farmed out to
auntie or grandma or, alternatively, taken along to work. In yet others,
they were left at home on their own or with siblings, without parental
support and with the unsettling prospect of having to manage by themselves in the event of an alarm.

With or without a parent, children were generally stuck indoors for
most of the day. In our discussion of the impact of the war on the family
(see Chapter 3), we described how this self-internment affected adults.
For children it meant relative isolation, protracted boredom, and lack of
sustaining structure. We already noted that Israeli children ordinarily
spend a considerable amount of time outdoors and go freely to friends'

homes. The country's clement climate, the low rate of street crime, and the organization of neighborhoods into fairly cohesive communities allow children a great deal of independent movement. In ordinary times, even first graders play on the street or the neighborhood park without parental supervision, walk or bike to after-school clubs on their own, and visit casually with friends without being dropped off or picked up by an adult. The ongoing missile threat put an abrupt end to these happy liberties. The community centers and clubs where children usually congregated shut their doors. People were wary of spending too much time outdoors, away from a sealed room. Even visiting with friends became problematic, as parents tended to be reluctant both to burden others with the care of an additional child in the event of an alarm and to take that responsibility on themselves.

The upshot was hours spent in front of the television, the tedium and tension of unstructured time, and the lack of release for pent-up energies (Lavie, D., 1991, p. 1). One of the questions posed to the staffers of the Ministry of Education hotline was how to pass the time when all the games were played, the books read, and the pictures drawn (Kachlili, 1991). The fact that such days followed upon nights when children were awakened by sirens and their sleep interrupted by sojourns in the sealed rooms added fatigue to these stresses.

The schools were reopened three weeks into the war. By this time, the pattern of nighttime attacks and daytime calm had become fairly established, and the expectation of chemical attack was reduced. The school authorities had the necessary plastic sheeting taped on the large schoolroom windows, and the school shelters were prepared for gas as well as conventional attack. The reopening of the school gates signaled a welcome return to some semblance of order and routine. It kept the children occupied and gave them a chance to be with their friends once again and to share their fears. Nonetheless, as emphasized by Dr. Josph Calev, director of the Children's Psychiatric Service of Ichilov Hospital in Tel Aviv, it was not a return to normalcy (Klausner, 1991). Teachers had to deal with the fatigue and lack of concentration of children awakened by nighttime alarms. Lessons were punctuated by shelter and gas mask drills. Recesses were staggered so that too many children would not be outside in the schoolyard at the same time. In the hallways sat parents on call to help out in case of an alarm. And the cumbersome gas masks were ubiquitous reminders of the lurking threat.

Moreover, even with the schools reopened, children still faced personal problems, such as the difficulty, in some families, of having to cope with parents who were visibly frightened and stressed (Bar-Yoseph, 1991). In more extreme cases, children were forced to take responsibility for highly distressed adults or to cope with parents who refused to wear their masks or go into the sealed room. Complaints to this effect were recorded by the Ministry of Education hotline (Noy, B., 1991).

Special problems arose for a small group of children who were in state-run facilities that were closed for all or part of the war. The journalist Judith Knoller (1991a) tells of what happened to children who were forced to leave a shelter run by the Ministry of Labor and Welfare and sent back to homes where they had suffered physical or sexual abuse. Some were thrown out and left to wander the streets or to be taken in by kindly neighbors. Some were subjected again to the abuse on account of which they had been removed from their homes in the first place. Others had to prepare the sealed room and otherwise take care of both themselves and their nonfunctioning parents. When the shelter was reopened a month into the war, many of the children returned in a state of emotional regression. Although these are the exceptions, and most children were certainly better taken care of, their plight shows what happens to the most vulnerable children when the strains on a country reduce the capacity and will of its institutions to take care of them.

The question addressed in this chapter, a variation of the questions asked in the other chapters, is how the special combination of stresses produced by the Gulf War affected the children who went through it. Research on children's responses to war has been much sparser on the whole than the study of adult responses. Klingman (1992) attributes the disparity to the methodological, ethical, and practical problems entailed in studying children, including such special difficulties as obtaining parental consent and permission to enter schools.

Moreover, very little of the research that has been carried out is applicable to the questions raised by the Gulf War. Terr (1985) has pointed out that the American, British, and French studies carried out in the 1940s on children in wartime focused on the parent–child relationship and the youngsters' responses to separation. Anna Freud's and Dorothy Burlingham's (1943) pioneering *War and Children*, for example, dealt almost entirely with English youngsters' reactions to being separated from their families. The studies explored the effects of temporary parental loss on children rather than the effects of war as such.

According to Terr (1985), children's reactions to traumatic events were not considered autonomous responses of their own but rather reflections of the responses of the surrounding adults (Despert, 1942). The few studies that did assess children's behavior in response to the air raids and bombardments in World War II (for example, Bordman, 1944; Brander, 1943) concluded, in the main, that chronic behavioral and psychological disturbances rarely resulted. Janis (1951), in keeping with the accepted view of the time, argued that the symptoms of acute anxiety that did arise could be traced to the emotional upset displayed by the children's parents.

Studies carried out on children in Israel are closer to home both geographically and in the types of war-related situations that gave rise to them, but their results are mixed and open to interpretation. Some also seem to provide evidence that children are resilient and do not develop significant long-term pathology in response to the dangers of war. For example, Ziv and Israeli's (1973) comparison of manifest anxiety scores of 10-year-old children living on seven kibbutzim along the Jordanian border that were under almost constant shelling at the time of the testing with those of children from seven kibbutzim that had never come under attack showed that the scores of the two groups were similar and uniformly low. Similarly, Milgram and Miller's (1973) comparison of 11-year-old children living in moshavim (cooperative farms) on the Jordanian border that were exposed to terrorist attack with their age-mates on unexposed moshavim in the center of the country found no group differences in manifest anxiety. This study even found that the children in the exposed communities displayed a higher level of personal autonomy and were more confident of their ability to overcome obstacles, to function independently of their parents, and to handle potentially frightening situations on their own. The findings of these studies may be particularly relevant because, unlike the World War II studies, they actually focused on children's responses to the life threat of war rather than on separation. These studies are of particular interest, since the stressors to which the kibbutz children were exposed were quite similar to those of the Gulf War, albeit more prolonged. In both cases, there was repeated exposure to intermittent shelling at night, a restriction of play and other recreational activities, and disruption of normal routines, though more so during the Gulf War. Moreover, the fact that the men of the house did not leave for the front made the situation investigated even more closely analogous to that of the Gulf War.

However, the kibbutzim and moshavim where those children lived are communal settlements very different from the towns and cities in which most Israelis make their homes. Ziv and Israeli (1973) explain the absence of observed differences in their study by the strong social cohesion and ideology of the kibbutz in those years and the intensive social support available to kibbutz children. Milgram and Miller (1973) suggest that the moshavim offered the children of their study similar supports. Thus, both studies leave open the question of whether children in noncohesive urban communities would survive the life threat of attack with similar equanimity.

In fact, studies carried out on children in Israel's cities and development towns (poorer, less culturally integrated towns in underdeveloped areas of the country) paint a less sanguine picture. Ziv, Kruglanski, and

Shulman (1974) found that following 18 months' calm, 8- to 14-year-olds who had previously been exposed to shelling showed more covert (but not overt) aggression than those who had not. Kristal (1978) found that while exposed and nonexposed 10- to 12-year-olds did not show differences in manifest anxiety following two years of calm, the former reported higher anxiety than the latter following a film simulating an attack on their settlement, suggesting, in the words of Chimienti, Nasr, and Khalifeth (1989), "sensitization of the exposed group to later stressful experiences" (p. 282). Other studies showed an increase of children's anxiety during and after the Yom Kippur War. Zak (1982) found an increase in anxiety traits and a decrease in certainty about how best to satisfy their needs among a group of high school seniors one year after the 1973 Yom Kippur War. Ziv (1975) reported a temporary increase of anxiety among Israeli children during wartime. Milgram and Milgram (1976) found the general anxiety scores of fifth- and sixth-grade urban children to be substantially higher during wartime than peacetime. On the other hand, Rofe and Lewin (1982) found that adolescents from a border town that sustained many years of intermittent shelling reported fewer daydreams about the tragic consequences of war and fewer aggressive daydreams about the enemy than their counterparts from a similar town that had not been shelled; were more compromising in their attitudes toward the Arabs; and, at night, fell asleep more quickly, slept longer, and reported fewer horror-filled dreams. However, they attribute these salutary findings to successful repression. One may question whether the development of a repressive personality style to deal with the threats of war is an entirely desirable outcome.

Findings on children's responses to other types of traumas similarly show vulnerability. Lacey (1972) found posttraumatic play and posttraumatic fears among 56 children who applied for counseling over a six-year period following a slag avalanche that had engulfed their primary school in Wales. Newman (1976) found a modified sense of reality, increased vulnerability to future stress, an altered sense of the power of the self, and earlier awareness of fragmentation and death among child survivors of the Buffalo Creek Flood. Pynoos et al. (1987) found that 40% of 159 elementary schoolchildren who survived a sniper attack in their school playground displayed moderate to severe posttraumatic stress disorder (PTSD) approximately one month after the event. At the 14-month follow-up, Nader, Pynoos, Fairbanks, and Fredrick (1990) reported that 74% of the children who had been trapped in the playground still showed moderate to severe PTSD. In an in-depth study of 26 schoolchildren who had been kidnapped at gunpoint from their schoolbus and buried alive for 16 hours, Terr (1983) found that four years after the event virtually all of them exhibited a large range of posttraumatic effects, which included pessimism about the future, belief in omens, memories of incorrect perceptions, thought suppression, shame, fear of reexperiencing traumatic anxiety, trauma-specific and mundane fears, posttraumatic play, behavioral reenactment, repetition of psychophysiological disturbances that began with the kidnapping, repeated nightmares, and a sense of a foreshortened future. More recently, Yule and Williams (1990) concluded that most of the 13 children they assessed who had survived the capsize of a British ferry in Zeebrugge harbor suffered from acute adjustment reactions that lasted upward of a year as well as from presenting symptoms that justified the diagnosis of PTSD. In another study of child survivors of this and other shipping disasters, Yule (1991) reported an array of stress symptoms. The problem with applying these findings of emotional damage to the children of the Gulf War is that the level of exposure was very different. The children in these disasters all suffered substantial personal harm or saw other people killed or seriously injured. Most of the children in the Gulf War were only threatened.

The aim of this chapter is to examine the impact of the Gulf War on Israeli children. The studies presented below use a systematic, empirical approach to measure a variety of immediate and longer-term responses among children of various ages. Most of them also explore factors that might mediate the impact of war on their subjects—shielding the children from possible emotional damage, on the one hand, or increasing their vulnerability, on the other.

It is worth pointing out that a relatively large number of studies on children have come out of the Gulf War, despite the short duration of the hostilities and the numerous and oft-noted methodological problems of researching children. This is a reflection of the relative technical ease of accessing children for study in Israel, where parents and the authorities in charge tend to be cooperative and children can be easily tested in their schools. More essentially, it reflects the intense concern with children in this country.

## EMPIRICAL STUDIES

### Infants, Toddlers, and Preschoolers

Of all age groups among children, the responses of the very young to war and other disasters have been the least studied. This may have to do with the difficulty of assessing adequate numbers of children who are too young to speak or to fill in questionnaires, as well as the need to rely heavily on the observations of parents, whose objectivity and accuracy are inevitably in question both because of their lack of professional training and, even more, because of their emotional involvement with their children. It is certainly very difficult to be sure that the parents are not projecting their own anxieties on their children or, on the other hand, as Yule (1991) and Terr (1985) suggest, underestimating their children's distress in an effort to deny traumatization.

Nonetheless, the issue of the impact of war on the very young is of great interest from both a practical and theoretical point of view. Theoretically, the question is whether their emotional and cognitive immaturity shields them from its adverse effects, because they cannot grasp or anticipate the dangers, or makes them more vulnerable, because they lack the defenses and other resources to cope with the threat. Practically, the question is of import because these children are at the age when their basic representations are formed, and any impact may be formative and enduring.

Two studies that we know of explored the responses of the very young to the Gulf War. The first suggests that the war had no more impact on the very young than it did on adults. The second shows a more complex dynamic of distress and coping, habituation, and exacerbation of distress.

### Sound Sleep

The simpler of the two studies was carried out by Lavie, Amit, Epstein, and Tzischinsky (1992) on infants' sleep. In what had begun as a more general study, the sleep habits and sleep disturbances of 61 infants were assessed by questionnaires completed by their parents five months before and one to two weeks after the war. No significant change was found in sleep habits or sleep quality.

The researchers also monitored the sleep of 55 infants using actigraphs, a monitor worn on the wrist at bedtime (see Chapter 2) during the last four weeks of the war. The data showed that although all the infants were awakened by the sirens, they went back to sleep immediately after the attack with no evidence of carryover effects.

On the whole, these findings are similar to those obtained in the same research laboratory on adults' sleep during the war, and are similarly at odds with the bulk of the research, which reports sleep difficulties in both children and adults.

### Vulnerability, Limited Habituation, and Coping Attempts

A much more detailed study was carried out by Rosenthal and Levy-Shiff (1993) on the initial and subsequent reactions of infants and toddlers (aged 4 to 36 months) to the war. This study has the virtue of honing in not only on general stress reactions but also on reactions to the major specific stressors of the war for young children: the gasproof tents that infants were placed in, the gas masks worn by older toddlers and their parents, the alarm, and the stay in the sealed room.

During the last two weeks of the war, semistructured interviews were administered to a sample of 99 mothers drawn, for comparison, from Scud-targeted Tel Aviv and a nontargeted area in Israel. Questions tapped specific responses to the alarms and safety precautions; general behaviors, including regressive conduct, adjustment disturbances, and changes in eating, sleeping, television watching and other habits; and various forms of coping activities both inside and outside the sealed room. Mothers were asked to rate their children both at the beginning of the war and at the time of the interview toward the end.

Results showed that many young children initially displayed very strong negative reactions to the "alarm state." Almost two-thirds (61.4%) reacted with crying, aggression, or fright at being placed in the gasproof tent or having their gas mask put on. Another 42.2% showed strong signs of distress simply at seeing their parents in masks. The sound of the siren upset 29.8%, and the stay in the sealed room upset 25%. On the other hand, a small percentage of the children showed cooperative behavior, such as climbing into the tents by themselves, handing their parents their gas masks to put on, bringing a bottle or pacifier for a younger sibling in the tent, and so forth. To the authors, these behaviors indicate their coping.

Results also showed signs of habituation similar to those displayed by older children and adults. About half of the children who were initially afraid to put on their masks and/or to see their parents in masks had become adjusted to these things by the war's end. On the other hand, a good proportion became increasingly distressed in the course of the war: about a third (36.3%) showed more intense responses to being placed in their sealed tents, and about a quarter (25.3%) found it more upsetting to see their parents in masks. Not surprisingly, those who showed the strongest distress in the early days of the war continued to show the strongest distress toward the war's end. These findings suggest something of the limits of habituation.

The limits of habituation are also suggested by the behavioral changes the mothers reported. On the one hand, some children became more helpful and cooperative (in matters not directly related to the masks and tents), and around half came to cope by play and humor on war-related themes. However, more than half (53.7%) showed changes in their usual eating and sleeping habits; more than half responded with adjustment difficulties such as prolonged crying, stomachaches, or temper tantrums (57.7%); and a small percentage regressed to less mature patterns of behavior (11.6%). Again, those who showed the greatest adjustment difficulties were the ones who had had the most intense emotional reactions to the sirens in the initial stages of the war.

The study also examined the impact of the children's age, their parents' responses to the war, and their geographic proximity to the target zone.

*Age.* The authors found that older toddlers reacted more strongly but adjusted more quickly than infants and younger toddlers. Older toddlers were found to display more intense emotional responses to the sealed room and more habit changes over time than their juniors. But, over time, they were less likely to show adjustment disturbances, coped better with the siren and the stay in the sealed room, and were more helpful to their family. As expected, they were more likely to engage in war-related play and to entertain their families with "witty jokes."

*Parents' Responses.* Children's reactions were also found to be related to those of their parents. Children whose mothers reported that the family showed intense distress reactions were, according to their mothers, less cooperative and helpful. Children whose mothers reported feeling that they needed help had, according to their mothers, more adjustment difficulties. On the other hand, children whose mothers reported coping well also seemed to cope better.

These associations are consistent with the widely held view discussed above that children's reactions to war are by and large reflections of their parents' reactions. The authors point out, however, that the correlations were rather weak and, moreover, that the direction of causality was not entirely certain: the children's distress and adjustment problems may have exerted pressure on the parents and intensified their distress as well as the other way around. The authors maintain that specific stresses such as the alarm state and the changes in daily routines that were part and parcel of the war for almost all families (92.7%) made their own independent contribution to the children's stress reactions.

*Proximity.* Findings showed that significantly more of the children in the target zone for Scud attacks changed their habits and routines and showed adjustment disturbances than children who resided in missile-free areas. Similarly, families residing in the target zone reported more immediate difficulties (such as uncertainty and unpredictability of the next moment, inability to leave the house, uncooperative children) and anticipated more difficulties in resuming their interrupted routines after the war. The effect of proximity on children was mediated by its effect on their parents.

The authors summarize their findings by pointing out that even very young children are vulnerable to war-related stressors but also manifest rudimentary attempts at coping. The findings also support the accepted role of parents as mediators of the impact of war on children, but give reason to believe that the specific stressors themselves are relevant. In addition, we may emphasize that age played a highly significant role in this group of very young children. Apparently, even the limited increase in maturity enabled the toddlers to cope better in the long run than the infants.

## Anxiety and Habituation in School-Age Children

Michael Rosenbaum and Tammie Ronen (1992) of Tel Aviv University examined anxiety levels in 277 fifth- and sixth-graders in two Tel Aviv public schools and their parents. In a three-way assessment, each child and his or her parents were asked to rate his or her own and the other two family members' anxiety levels on a 10-point scale. They were asked to make these ratings for six distinct times in the course of the day: morning, evening, night, at the sound of the alarm, while they were in the sealed room, and immediately after leaving the sealed room. The study was conducted during the fifth week of the war, and the participants were asked to rate both their current anxiety and, retrospectively, their anxiety during the first week of the war.

In both the first and last weeks of the war, children's self-reported anxiety levels stood between those of their mothers and their fathers. During the daytime, their anxiety levels were closer to the lower level of their fathers; at night they approached the higher level of their mothers. The one exception was in the sealed room, when the anxiety level of boys was identical to that of the grown men. Throughout, girls reported a somewhat higher level of anxiety than boys, but the difference did not reach significance. Examination of correlations within families revealed that the children's self-reported anxiety levels generally correlated somewhat with those of their mothers, but not at all with those of their fathers.

Children's anxiety levels fluctuated much like those of their parents, being higher at night than during the day, and highest at the sound of the alarm and in the sealed room. Since all but one of the Scud attacks took place at night, the anxiety levels corresponded to the times of danger. Moreover, also like their parents, children reported considerably less anxiety during the fifth week of the war than during the first.

This is yet further evidence of the habituation or accommodation demonstrated in Chapter 2 on the general population.

The three-way assessment enabled the authors to examine the correspondence between the way children viewed their anxiety and the ways in which their parents saw it. In general, there was a moderate degree of correspondence between the children's self-reports of their anxiety and the parents' perceptions of it, especially in the sealed room, when families were together. Mothers, however, tended to view their children as more anxious than fathers did.

Klingman (1992) also found a pattern of habituation in the 7th-, 10th-, and 12th-grade pupils whose stress symptoms he examined during the first and fourth weeks of the war. The assessment was made in two areas, one high-risk, the other low-risk. In both groups, the most frequent stress-related symptoms the first week were fear of being hit by a missile (69%), curtailment of enjoyable activities (59%), and difficulty in falling asleep following an alarm (58%). Other responses included overeating (49%), physical weakness (48%), concentration difficulties (48%), sleep disturbances (43%), restlessness (35%), and physical pain (31%). From these percentages, one can see that a good proportion of the youngsters endorsed symptoms. However, in the course of the war, the endorsement of symptoms declined in both groups from a mean of 5.8 in the first week to 3.0 by the fourth.

Klingman also found that symptoms differed with the age, gender, and exposure of the children. During both the first and last weeks of the war, the seventh graders endorsed more physical pains, frightening dreams, and undereating than the 10th and 12th graders. Girls reported a higher frequency of stress reactions than boys. And children from the high-risk areas reported a significantly greater frequency of some symptoms (such as curtailment of pleasant activities, the presence of physical pains, and feelings of restlessness) than those from the low-risk areas.

Along similar lines, Mintz (1992) examined anxiety levels and physiological symptoms in 313 7th- and 10th-grade children from high- and low-risk areas. This study had the advantage of using a standardized measure of anxiety: the Spielberger State-Trait Anxiety Inventory. Results are consistent with those of Klingman. The younger adolescents reported higher levels of anxiety than the older teenagers. Girls showed more anxiety than boys. Children in both 7th and 10th grades who lived closer to the attacked areas reported higher levels of anxiety than those living in less attacked areas.

These three studies make a number of overlapping points:

1. All show a certain level of distress among children.
2. Two of them, Rosenbaum and Ronen's and Klingman's (1992),

indicate a process of habituation among children similar to that found in the babies studied by Rosenthal and Levy-Shiff (1993) and in the adult population discussed in Chapter 2. In this process, a portion of the children apparently became accustomed to the various stresses and reacted with less distress, whereas others were still experiencing notable distress at the end of February. The mothers' reports in the telephone survey suggest that, the habituation notwithstanding, there might have been a long-term residual effect.

3. Two studies, Klingman's (1992) and Mintz's (1992), point to three risk factors: (1) Degree of exposure, in terms of proximity to the missile attacks, was related to the amount of distress, with children in high-risk areas registering more distress than those in low-risk areas. (2) Gender proved to play a significant role in the amount of anxiety the children displayed, with girls showing more than boys. (3) Age was a significant factor in children's responses to the war, with younger adolescents (12- to 13-year-olds) manifesting greater distress than older ones.

## Responses to the War and Possible Antecedents in School-Age Children

### An Increase in Common Childhood Symptoms

Ronen and Rahav (1991) attempted to gauge the distress of school-age children by comparing the frequency of symptoms of emotional problems three weeks into the war with the frequency before the war. The subjects were 157 second and 159 sixth graders in a large Tel Aviv primary school. Shortly after the schools were reopened, the children filled out a self-report symptom frequency questionnaire consisting of 15 common childhood symptoms of distress (for example, nail biting, sleep disturbance). Every child answered the questionnaire twice: once with regard to his or her current wartime symptoms and once with regard to symptoms three months earlier.

The major finding was of a significant increase, averaging 43%, in the number of stress symptoms reported by children in both grades during the war. The three most frequently reported symptoms during the war—nail biting, headaches, and sleep disorders—were also the symptoms reported to be most frequent before the war. However, 12 out of the 15 symptoms were more prevalent during than before the war, though relatively small percentages of children reported decreases in one or another of the symptoms. In particular, there were substantial increases in reports of sleep disorders, nightmares, nonspecific pains, and headaches. Enuresis (bedwetting) was one of the least frequent symptoms to begin with. On the whole, the second graders seem to have endorsed a somewhat higher frequency of most of the symptoms than the sixth graders. In the matter of bedwetting the difference reached statistical significance.

Gender did not make a significant contribution to the number of wartime problem behaviors, though second-grade boys endorsed more nonspecific aches than second-grade girls, and sixth-grade girls endorsed more stomachaches, teeth grinding, and headaches than sixth-grade boys. The authors explain the lack of gender difference, which has been found in so many other studies, by the relatively young age of the subjects and/or by the fact that since behaviors were studied, they were not subject to the known gender differences in willingness to report emotions.

The number of prewar problems a child reported was found to be the best predictor of the number of wartime problems. In both age groups children with an above-average level of prewar behavioral problems displayed a greater increase in problems during the war than children with fewer behavioral problems before the war. In particular, second graders with a large number of prewar problem habits showed an especially high frequency of such problems during the war. This finding supports the view that pretrauma psychological functioning affects children's responses to traumatic events.

On the other hand, the authors also noted that when they looked at the specific changes among children who endorsed having had a particular symptom before the war and those who had not endorsed that symptom, they found that a higher proportion of children seemed to have lost or dropped bad habits than acquired a new bad habit. They emphasize that these data show that changes produced by stress are "by no means unidirectional."

Moreover, summing up their findings, they point out that both the kind and reported frequency of the wartime problems remained within what is often described as the normal range for children of similar ages. They also offer the disclaimer that because of the very low rate of such problems to begin with, the measurement of changes was subject to floor and ceiling effects.

### Anxiety, Coping, and Personal Resources: A Semiprojective Picture Test for Children

Zeidner, Klingman, and Itskovitz (1993) attempted to investigate the relationships between children's personal and social resources and their coping and affective reactions during the war. Subjects were 170 fourth and fifth graders drawn from three middle-class neighborhood schools situated in three cities at different levels of risk for missile attack: Ramat Gan, which sustained the most missile attacks and the heaviest Scud damage; Haifa, where there were fewer attacks; and Tiberias, outside the missile trajectory.

In March, right after the end of the war, the children completed an adaptation of the semiprojective Bar Ilan Picture Test for Children (Itskovitz & Strauss, 1982) in groups in their home rooms at school. The version used in the study consists of six pictures of children and their parents, teachers, and friends in different home and school situations. Each situation was adapted to fit he Gulf War and accompanied by projective questions. For example, the first picture depicted a typical school route accompanied by the following instructions: "The children are on their way to school after a missile attack at night, and they are talking about their experience. What does the girl say to the boy? What does the boy say in response? What will they do in school? What will they do if there's another alert?" On the basis of their answers, the children were each rated on 20 items that ranged over the two outcome measures, namely their anxiety and coping during the war, and the various resources deemed to affect those outcomes, including their perceived control over the wartime situation, perceived social support, the quality of their defenses, and their verbal and emotional expressiveness.

Findings showed that almost all the children projected feelings of fear and anxiety (89%) and that around a third expressed loneliness (35%) and sadness (31%). On the other hand, relatively few gave voice to the more extreme feelings of panic (23%), shame (17%), anger (8%), and confusion (8%). This distribution of responses is similar in nature to that recorded by adults (see Chapter 2), with most of the feelings in the manageable range and the very strong and disruptive feelings decidedly minority phenomena.

Along similar lines, most of the children (63%) were rated as projecting a moderate sense of control over the situation, while a sizable minority projected a sense of helplessness (29%), and a tiny fraction a sense of omnipotence (3%). Most of them also described the parental figures in the pictures as supportive (fathers 63% and mothers 58%), while a similarly large minority described them as worried (29% for fathers and mothers both) and lesser numbers as pressured (22% and 15%), needing help (13% and 6%), and/or angry (9% and 12%). The defense mechanisms projected onto the figures included intellectualization (42%), denial (38%), projection (32%), reaction formation (13%), isolation (11%), and regression (9%).

Coping and anxiety were found to have a moderate inverse relationship to one another, though when other variables were controlled for, coping did not make a unique contribution to anxiety. Moreover, both coping and anxiety were found to be related to the internal and external resources the children brought to the war. The children who were rated as effective copers were also rated as having high perceived control, high perceived social support, and more complex defenses and better verbal skills than poorer copers. Put in terms of how the variables were operationalized, the better copers conveyed the feeling that something could be done to handle the stressful encounters (control), and they described the parental figures in the pictures as supportive and the families as communicating well (support). The children who were rated as less anxious similarly conveyed greater perceived control and more effective defenses than those who were more anxious, and they also perceived the parental figures as somewhat less anxious.

To some extent, these findings are tautological, in that effective defenses were operationalized as defenses that reduced anxiety. However, the finding of interrelations between the children's coping and anxiety, on the one hand, and the resources at their disposal, on the other, is generally in keeping with other findings in the literature on stress. As the authors document, sense of control, social support, and effective defenses have all been shown to mediate stress and facilitate coping (Lazarus & Folkman, 1984). Moreover, the moderate correlation between the anxiety of the children and that which they attributed to the parental figures in the pictures accords with the moderate correlation found by Rosenthal and Levy-Shiff (1993) between the level of parental distress and the level of the distress of the infants and toddlers they studied. This correlation is further evidence that while parents may filter war and other stressful experiences for their children, they are neither the single nor necessarily decisive factor in children's reactions.

However, of all the studies that examined the effect of degree of exposure on children, this was the only one to find no significant association between the respondents' psychological distress and their proximity to the missile target areas. No difference was found in the anxiety levels of the children in heavily attacked Tel Aviv, moderately attacked Haifa, and unattacked Tiberias. A possible explanation might be that by the time this study was undertaken, a month after the war's end, any earlier differences were canceled out. The study conducted by the Israel Institute for Military Studies discussed in Chapter 2 similarly found that fear responses among adults evened out in heavily scudded Tel Aviv, less scudded Haifa, and nonstricken Zikhron Ya'akov (Gal R., 1991).

Indeed, under the circumstances of the war, the external validity of the adapted version of the measure that was used was never established, though it was established for the original picture test. Thus Zeidner,

Klingman, and Itskovitz (1993) caution that "the data reflect how the children responded to the test and not (necessarily) how they behaved when the missile danger was imminent" (p. 27) and warn that "the 'anxiety' and 'coping' displayed in the subjects' responses to the pictures must not be interpreted as retrospective indications of their actual feelings and conduct in the crisis." Among other possibilities, it seems to us that the data might better reflect the short-term psychological sequelae of the war: the feelings of anxiety and mastery with which children were left.

## EMOTIONAL SEQUELAE OF THE WAR

Several researchers undertook to examine the emotional sequelae of the war. Three of the studies presented below looked at the residues of the war within a few months of its end; one followed up the impact a year later as well.

### Stress Evaporation and Stress Residuals

Raviv and Raviv (1991) summarized two telephone surveys conducted by the Dahaf Research Institute four and six months after the war. In the first, the 237 parents who participated reported greater fear among younger children (under 14) than among adolescents (over 14) and a marked decrease in fear over the four months since the war, which suggests an evaporation of wartime stress.

In the second survey, the 366 parents who participated reported greater fear in their children during the war than in the survey two months earlier. This difference points up the unreliability of parental assessment of the children. It may be attributed to changes in parents' own recall of the war. My personal impression is that with the war's end people wanted to put its tensions out of mind. It was only about half a year later, when the anxieties were perhaps worked through somewhat, that they felt free to recollect and acknowledge them.

### The Gulf War and the Intifada

Greenbaum, Erlich, and Toubiana (1992) tried to examine the impact of living with the Intifada, the Palestinian uprising in the West Bank and Gaza, on children's reactions to the Gulf War several months later. The Intifada had been going on the three years before the outbreak of the Gulf War and was still going strong when the study was carried out in

May and June 1991. Conceptually, the authors' aim was to ascertain whether exposure to long-term stress (the Intifada) affects responses to a relatively short, time-limited stressor (the Gulf War).

To this end they compared the responses of 150 Jewish fifth to eighth graders living in the West Bank to those of an analogous population of 278 children form the Jerusalem area via questionnaires administered in their classrooms. Neither of the areas in question sustained any war damage, and both were considered especially safe. The two groups differed in that the children from the territories had lived with an overhanging threat of violence for the previous three years, while the Jerusalem children had not. The West Bank children were in constant danger of rocks and molotov cocktails being thrown at their school buses and parents' cars, which in some cases had resulted in the physical injury and even death of other children and adults living in the settlements. The Jerusalem group shared few of these experiences.

The researchers found that the children in both groups were less concerned with the Gulf War than with current matters. They were most concerned with traffic accidents and, on a lower level, with their schoolwork and relationships with friends. Their concern with the Gulf War was similar in intensity to their concern with school and friends. The only area where the two groups differed significantly was in their ratings of the Intifada, about which the West bank children naturally expressed more concern than the Jerusalem group. In short, the study did not show that the children who had been exposed to the long-term stress of the Intifada were more troubled or affected by the Gulf War than children who had not been so exposed.

The authors interpret these findings as indicating that once a highly salient threatening event passes, other items in the child's agenda resume their traditional importance. For the West Bank children, these items obviously included the Intifada, whose threat was still very potent while that of the Gulf War was not. A study conducted during or immediately after the war might have shown different results. What does seem to be of relevance here is that even several months after the missile attacks had come to an end, the war remained as much a matter of concern to all the children as their schoolwork and friends, which are no slight matters.

Interestingly, the authors found gender differences in the responses of the children from both groups. Girls, especially those from the territories, scored higher than boys in worry about both the Intifada and the Gulf War. On the other hand, there was no difference between the sexes in overall anxiety and coping scores, and boys from both Jerusalem and the territories gave more Intifada-related responses to some words (especially "tire" and "collaborator") in a word association test. In the view of the authors, the boys' lower reports of stress may be due to their greater use than girls of response repression and denial in coping with fear and anxiety.

## Anticipated Willingness to Serve in the Army

Moshe Israelshvili (1992) attempted to assess the impact of the Gulf War on the willingness of high schoolers to serve in the army in the near future. The readiness of the country's youth to serve is an important issue in Israel at any time. After the Gulf War, the author was concerned that the danger to the home front and the fact that no fighting took place would create a conflict for young Israelis; that is, they would be caught between their basic readiness to serve in the military and their natural desire to be with their families and protect them in time of trouble. To test this hypothesis, Israelshvili surveyed 954 11th and 12th graders in five Tel Aviv high schools, all of them in areas where missiles actually fell. The survey was conducted in the course of the war itself, between January 24 and February 14. It queried both the students' current feeling and their anticipated readiness to do their military duty in the near future.

Over 60% reported that they were at least moderately distressed and fearful in the wake of the missile attacks, but a good three-quarters were confident that they could cope with another round. Both their fear and confidence in their coping ability were significantly associated with the example of family and friends. Those who reported that their parents and schoolmates coped and functioned well tended to report less fear and distress and greater confidence in their ability to cope with future attacks. Very few (8%) were willing to talk to a school counselor or a psychologist, which suggests that most students either did not need or were unwilling to ask for professional help. Those willing to do so, however, tended to be self-confident young people who believed that they commanded the respect of their teachers.

The main finding of the study was that 32% of the young people queried reported that they were more willing to serve in the IDF as a result of the Gulf War, while only 4% said that they felt less willing than before. The national emergency apparently increased rather than decreased young people's readiness to do their military duty. On the other hand, the approximately 20% of the responded who reported high levels of distress during the war expressed less readiness to serve than those who felt easier. In the author's view, this means that a greater threat to the civilian population in the future could seriously reduce young people's willingness to serve in the army. One may question this prediction, however. The study looked at anticipated, not actual, readiness to serve. Such reluctance may be short-lived.

## One Month After and One Year Later

A large study that specifically addresses the psychological sequelae of the traumatic stress of the war among children was conducted by my colleagues and myself (Schwarzwald, Weisenberg, Solomon, & Waysman, in press; Schwarzwald, Weisenberg, Waysman, Solomon, & Klingman, 1993; Weisenberg, Schwarzwald, Waysman, Solomon, & Klingman, 1993). The study was carried out in two phases, the first at the end of March 1991, about a month after the cessation of fighting, and the second a year later in March 1992. Both parts focus on the contribution of various objective and subjective factors to the children's reactions.

## PART I: STRESS, COPING, AGE, AND GENDER: ANTECEDENTS OF DISTRESS

The first part of the study tried to determine the extent to which the children's level of distress immediately after the war was a function of (1) the intensity of the stress they experienced during the war, (2) their coping strategies in the sealed room, (3) their age, and (4) their gender. The children's emotional responses in the sealed room were also examined.

A battery of questionnaires was administered in their classrooms to a total of 492 Israeli children from the 5th (age 10–11), 7th (age 12–13), and 10th (age 15–16) grades in two cities: Tel Aviv, which had sustained 17 missile strikes during the war, and Natanya, which had sustained none.

The intensity of stress during the war was gauged by both objective and subjective measures. The objective measure consisted of (1) proximity to the sites where the missiles fell and (2) the physical damage caused by the strikes both directly to the child and his or her home and indirectly to relatives, friends, and acquaintances. The subjective measure asked the respondents to rate the degree of danger that they had believed they, their family, their friends, and their homes were in.

Emotional reactions and coping activities in the sealed room were measured by a specially designed questionnaire consisting of 41 items—16 tapping emotional responses and 25 tapping coping efforts. The children were asked to rate the extent to which each item characterized their reactions or behavior in the sealed room on a 3-point scale: not at all, a little, or a lot.

Stress after the war was assessed by the Stress Reaction Questionnaire made up of 20 items based on the Frederick and Pynoos (1988) Child Posttraumatic Stress Reaction Index interview and 6 items derived from the DSM-III-R diagnostic criteria for posttraumatic stress disorder (PTSD). The latter were added to permit a structured assessment of clinical-level PTSD. Examples of items are "I get scared when I think about the war," "Since the war, I've had more headaches, stomachaches, or other pains," and "Since the war, I do things that I did when I was younger but had stopped doing (such as sucking my thumb or sleeping with a teddy bear)." Children were asked to rate each item of a 3-point scale: not at all, a little, or a lot.

Most of the children reported feeling tense in the sealed room (75.8%). At the same time, most of them also endorsed positive emotions such as being confident that everything would be OK (80%) and feeling relaxed (78.2%). Only a much smaller, though substantial, proportion admitted to somatic effects such as trembling (51.7%), sweating (31%), stomachaches (32%), and headaches (44.5%). And an even smaller proportion endorsed more extreme expressions of tension such as crying (17.4%) and the feeling that they would go crazy (17.8%).

On the surface, these endorsements seem contradictory. It is difficult to grasp how over three-quarters of the children could endorse both having felt tense and having felt relaxed. One interpretation is that denial played heavily in these children's defenses. Virtually all the other studies that looked into the matter found considerable apprehension in the sealed room. The children, like their elders, were in a passive, helpless position, uncertain as to whether a missile would strike the vicinity of their home and what kind of warhead it would carry. Like their parents, they were also glued to the television and radio reports of events, which made the threat all the more tangible. Given these factors, as well as the endorsement of somatic symptoms of stress by about a third to a half of the respondents, their positive feelings can be read as representing their efforts to isolate and encapsulate their fears.

At the same time, the same child may have been sometimes tense and sometimes relaxed, sometimes scared and sometimes optimistic about the outcome of the war (which is one of the highly endorsed coping devices; see below). This interpretation is in keeping with the extensive evidence of habituation, in that it would allow for the children to have calmed down as the war progressed. It is also logical that the same person may have had contradictory feelings. The instructions enabled the respondents to endorse either a little or a lot of each response, and even a small amount was calculated as an endorsement.

## Coping Responses

Like the emotional responses, a fair number of the coping strategies were also endorsed by an overwhelming majority of the children. These included following radio and television broadcasts (96.6%); distracting themselves by talking to the other people in the room (90.6%); monitoring by checking to see if everyone was OK (89.8%) and checking their gas masks (82.6%); helping (89.8%) and calming (85.4%) others; and engaging in wishful thinking such as wishing for a miracle (88.5%), wishing it was a false alarm (82.2%), and wishing that the missiles would fall elsewhere (81.2%). About three-quarters of the respondents also endorsed acting as though everything was as usual (74.2%)—which lends further support to the prevalence of denial.

## Emotion and Coping as Functions of Gender

Girls endorsed more tension, fear, crying, sense of isolation, stomachaches, headaches, and trembling than boys, and reported more that they were in constant fear that something would happen to them. Also, while boys tended to report more that they tried to calm down others in the sealed room, girls tended to report more that they asked their parents to hug them and that they telephoned friends or relatives.

## Postwar Distress and Wartime Stress

In general, children's stress responses one month after the war appeared to be contingent on both the objective and subjective stress they had suffered. Children who lived in parts of Tel Aviv that were hit by missiles and who were emotionally close to people who suffered missile damage endorsed both higher levels of subjective stress during the war and higher levels of distress after the war than those who were geographically and emotionally more distant from the threat.

Results also showed that 25% of the children living in the high-risk Tel Aviv area and 13% of those living in Natanya met DSM-III-R criteria for PTSD. Since PTSD is a clinical diagnosis, these rates indicate that the war left considerable psychological sequelae, at least in the short term. These sequelae were more extensive among the Tel Aviv children than those in the safer city of Natanya. This differentiation corresponds to other findings on the impact of proximity to a traumatogenic event.

However, a fair percentage of the children who lived outside the missile trajectory also suffered emotional damage from this frightening war with its ubiquitous, uncertain threat.

Teachers' appraisals partially validated the students' self-reports. Students whose classroom performance was rated as having deteriorated since the war had higher distress scores than those whose performance was rated as better or the same. Teachers also observed deterioration in academic functioning in 24% of the children diagnosed with PTSD and impairment in social functioning in 11% of the children with PTSD. Among those rated as showing a deterioration in intellectual functioning, 32% were categorized as suffering from PTSD, in comparison to only 18% of those not so categorized.

These appraisals can be interpreted in two ways. One is that the teachers were unable to perceive or reluctant to acknowledge these children's sufferings. This explanation has been put forward by Yule and Williams (1990) in their follow-up of children who survived a shipping disaster. There is a consensus in recent literature that teachers report less psychopathology among child survivors of disasters than do parents and that both report far less than the child victims themselves (Earls, Smith, Reich, & Jung, 1988; McFarlane, Policansky, & Irwin, 1987). The other interpretation is that the appraisals indicate that even children with pathological levels of emotional distress can continue to function on social and academic levels.

## Postwar Distress as a Function of Age

Age was a factor in both the nonclinical and clinical levels of distress, with younger children proving themselves more vulnerable. In general, 5th graders, especially girls, endorsed higher levels of distress than 7th and 10th graders (whose stress levels did not differ significantly) even though they did not subjectively perceive themselves as more vulnerable during the war. The 5th graders also showed the highest rates of PTSD—33%—followed by 14% of the 7th graders and 9% of the 10th graders. These findings suggest that preadolescents are more susceptible to the impact of traumatic events than adolescents, and that younger adolescents are more susceptible than older adolescents.

## Postwar Distress as a Function of Gender

Girls reported higher subjective stress during the war and showed more global symptoms after the war than their male counterparts. Moreover, of all the children, fifth-grade girls were the most likely to have PTSD.

## Wartime Coping and Postwar Distress

As expected, coping skill was related to the level of distress after the war. The children who suffered the most postwar psychological symptoms reported the most monitoring behaviors and the most reassurance-seeking (asking their parents to hug them and acting as if everything were as usual) in the sealed room. Along with the children who showed a moderate level of symptoms, they also used less verbal—or social—distraction than the low-symptom children. That is, they talked less to the other people in the room, and they did not release their tension by making fun of the situation, as those with less serious postwar residues did. Similarly, children with PTSD also did more checking, were more prone to seek reassurance, and made less use of verbal distraction than children without PTSD.

These findings suggest that certain coping strategies were more effective than others in moderating the adverse impact of stress. Monitoring was linked with higher levels of postwar distress than distraction and avoidance in the form of conversation and humor. To some extent, this distinction is consistent with other studies that show the limitations of problem-focused coping in situations that cannot be changed (Lazarus & Folkman, 1984). Under the circumstances at hand, once the room was sealed and the mask was on one's head, all further checking was pointless and rather frenetic.

At the same time, the opposite of active coping—denial in the form of behaving as if everything were as usual and emotion-focused coping in the form of asking to be hugged—was also linked to high postwar distress. The mixed results suggest that the distinction in the literature between active- and emotion-focused coping may not be adequate to explain the psychiatric residues of traumatic events and that more subtle distinctions are called for.

## Coping, Age, and Postwar Residues

The findings on coping are perhaps best understood in connection with the findings on age. Analysis of the relation between age and coping showed that children of different ages tended to cope differently. Fifth graders used significantly less interpersonal verbal distraction than 7th and 10th graders, but more of them asked to be hugged and acted as if everything were as usual; they also engaged in more pointless monitoring than 10th graders. At the same time, the 10th graders engaged in significantly more intrapersonal distraction (such as reading, or thinking about things unrelated to the war). Although the use of intrapersonal distraction did not contribute to the psychological outcome, it remains that the 5th graders tended to use less situationally effective coping strategies than the 7th and 10th graders.

The key seems to be the age-related cognitive ability to choose the right coping method in the situation. For example, the 10-year-olds' simple denial in the form of acting as if everything was as usual was less effective than more complex forms of avoidance, such as humor and conversation, of which the older children were capable. Similarly, the social support that the older children may have obtained through conversation seems to have been more effective than the social support that the younger children obtained through physical contact.

With all of this, it should be kept in mind that the findings are correlational. Another interpretation of them is that the choice of coping methods was itself affected by the amount of stress the children felt. Children who were more stressed during the war may have chosen less effective coping methods than those who were more stressed, and both their coping methods and their level of postwar stress were outcomes of the level of their wartime stress.

## PHASE II: LONG-TERM SEQUELAE

Of the children who had participated in the first phase of the investigation, 326 were studied again a year later. The follow-up sample contained a larger proportion of girls in the areas that had sustained missile strikes, but otherwise the two samples were similar. The attrition was not a function of the immediate postwar stress ratings that had been obtained, nor of grade level, nor of region or sex alone. Assessments were made using the same Stress Reaction Questionnaire that had been used in Phase I of the study, and the same procedure was employed. The one addition was that the children were also asked whether their home had been hit in any of the strikes and, if so, whether the damage had been repaired. This question was added under the assumption that children whose homes were hit and not repaired within the year would be the ones most likely to still show any residuals of the war at the time of the study.

The second phase was designed to assess the impact of time on responses to traumatic events and was conducted within the framework of two contrasting approaches to the subject: the stress evaporation perspective and the residual stress perspective. As its name suggests, the stress evaporation theory holds that stress reactions disappear over time (for example, Borus, 1973; Solomon, Weisenberg, Schwarzwald, & Mikulincer, 1987). The residual stress approach, in contrast, maintains that traumatic events can leave long-lasting emotional damage (for example, Figley, 1978; Strayer & Ellenhorn, 1975). As noted in the first part of this chapter, both views have found support in studies of children exposed to war.

The findings of the present study support both views. As can be seem from Table 5.1, general stress symptomatology declined dramatically from its level immediately after the war. On the other hand, as our regression analysis indicated, those who scored high right after the war also scored relatively high at the year's end. A similar pattern is discernible in PTSD status. Overall, the rate declined from 22.1% to 12.0% of the sample. Yet, while a good proportion of the children diagnosed with PTSD right after the war were no longer diagnosable as such at the end of the year, a fair number of children who had not had PTSD developed it.

As in the earlier study, age and proximity to damage both played a role. As can be seen from the table, a year after the war the greatest stress symptomatology was on the whole still recorded in the regions that had been hit. PTSD rates remained highest there as well. Furthermore, children whose homes had been hit showed significantly higher levels of general stress and significantly higher levels of PTSD than those whose homes had not been hit (23.8% versus 9.1%) though, contrary to expectations, their mental health was not influenced by whether or not their homes had been repaired. It was, however, influenced by their age. Among the children who did not have diagnosable PTSD at the end of

**Table 5.1. Means and Standard Deviations (in Parentheses) of General Stress Symptomatology Scores by Region, Grade, and Sex**

|  |  | Region hit | | Region not hit | |
|---|---|---|---|---|---|
| Sex | Grade | Phase I | Phase II | Phase I | Phase II |
| Males | Six | 22.26 | 16.46 | 18.36 | 11.00 |
|  |  | (12.58) | (11.95) | (8.85) | (9.36) |
|  | Eight | 12.10 | 6.50 | 8.67 | 5.80 |
|  |  | (8.40) | (5.27) | (8.18) | (5.29) |
|  | Eleven | 12.20 | 9.60 | 3.33 | 3.67 |
|  |  | (11.75) | (10.25) | (3.72) | (1.51) |
| Females | Six | 29.12 | 14.78 | 14.81 | 9.08 |
|  |  | (14.51) | (10.71) | (11.08) | (8.26) |
|  | Eight | 16.80 | 9.20 | 15.52 | 14.56 |
|  |  | (8.85) | (6.88) | (11.64) | (17.38) |
|  | Eleven | 16.92 | 10.31 | 11.57 | 7.79 |
|  |  | (10.45) | (9.20) | (7.71) | (6.26) |

the war, the 5th graders in the areas that had been hit by missiles developed significantly more delayed reactions than the 7th and 10th graders. Of those in the stricken area who did have PTSD, almost 40% of the fifth graders still had it at year's end, while none of the older children did.

In short, the findings suggest that the persistence of trauma effects depends on a conveyance of factors: the severity of the initial reaction, the degree of exposure, and the age of the child. While most of the children in this study soon recovered from any detrimental effects their war experience may have caused them, the stronger their initial distress, the younger their age, and the more intense their exposure, the more likely they were to show persistent long-term emotional damage. These were much the same factors that influenced the intensity of their immediate postwar response.

## DISCUSSION

Virtually all of the studies (excluding the Lavie et al., 1992, sleep study) showed that children of all ages, from infancy through late teens, experienced elevated levels of anxiety during the war. A minority of children showed indications of various degrees of morbidity, as manifested by the onset or increased frequency of stress-related behaviors during the war (Ronen & Rahav, 1991) and by war-induced PTSD afterward (Schwarzwald et al., 1993).

Nonetheless, the findings also show that most children were able to respond to the stress of the war adaptively, even in areas where missiles fell close to home. Despite the high level of threat and pervasive uncertainty, the external disorganization in their lives, the disruption of normal routines, and the loss of important sources of social support, most children coped. There was no more panic among children than there was among adults. Nor were there any published reports of reactive psychoses or epidemics of anxiety reactions among children. Social workers at a major Tel Aviv hospital even thought there was a decrease in the proportion of children brought to the emergency room, though it is difficult to know whether this was due to a special wartime effort on the part of children and their parents to handle problems on their own or to the temporary departure from Tel Aviv by a large number of families with children. Whichever the case, virtually all the studies that assessed responses over time showed that as the war wore on, most children, like most of the adults discussed in Chapter 2, showed a pattern of accommodation and reduced anxiety (Klingman, 1992; Rosen-

baum & Ronen, 1992; Rosenthal & Levy-Shiff, 1993). With the end of
the war, there seems to have been a fair degree of, though not total,
evaporation of stress responses. Studies carried out a month or so after
the war found discernible stress residues (Zeidner, Klingman & Itskovitz, 1993; Weisenberg, Schwarzwald, Waysman, Solomon, & Klingman,
1993; Schwarzwald, Weisenberg, Solomon, & Waysman, in press). But a
few months later, the war was no longer uppermost in children's concerns (Greenbaum, Erlich, & Toubiana, 1992). By a year later, as far as
can be determined from the one long-term study that was carried out
(Schwarzwald, et al., in press), many of the ill effects had evaporated.
Both general stress symptomatology and PTSD rates had significantly
declined.

To be sure, the studies also showed that in both the short and long
terms there were children who did not adapt. Rosenthal and Levy-Shiff
(1993) found an intensification of stress responses in the course of the
war among some of the very young children they studied. Schwarzwald
et al. (in press) found that a good number of the children who had PTSD
a month after the war still had it a year later and that some children even
developed delayed PTSD. However, the long-term PTSD was concentrated primarily among children in areas that had been hit by Scuds.

Thus, on the whole, the findings presented in this chapter indicate
that there was little significant damage to Israel's children in the Gulf
War. In part, this can be explained by Helson's (1964) account, three
decades ago, of the adaptation of Israeli kibbutz children to the shelling
with which they lived: "The shelling situation becomes, over time, part
of the children's way of life. They learn to deal with this stress situation
in a matter of fact, constructive way" (cited in Milgram, 1982a, p. 658).
Even babies and toddlers were shown to have developed rudimentary
modes of coping with the emergency situation (Rosenthal & Levy-Shiff,
1993).

More meaningfully, the absence of substantial emotional damage
can be explained by the nature of the Gulf War itself. The Gulf War was
truly frightening because of the overhanging life threat and ongoing
uncertainties. There were, however, almost no deaths or serious injuries,
and damage to home and property was highly contained. In contrast to
children caught up in other wars, Israeli children in the Gulf War were
not exposed to any of the horrors of fighting, as described for example
by Garbarino, Kostelny, and Dubrow (1991). They did not see dead or
mutilated bodies, did not lose family members, were not separated from
their parents and left to fend for themselves, and did not want for food
or shelter. They suffered neither the personal abuse that attends disasters caused by human beings nor the dislocation and havoc of natural

catastrophes. Most of them remained with their parents, enjoying the protection of their families, while the violence they saw was restricted largely to the television screen.

The studies reviewed here identified several factors that may have been associated with different levels of vulnerability among Israeli children during the Gulf War. These include exposure, age, gender, and prewar emotional problems.

## Level of Exposure

Several of the studies demonstrated that children with higher exposure to the missile attacks showed more anxiety and sustained more long-term damage. These included children from the frequently bombed city of Tel Aviv and, more specifically, children from neighborhoods that sustained missile damage. On the whole, Tel Aviv children of all ages (Klingman, in press; Mintz, 1992; Raviv & Raviv, 1992; Rosenthal & Levy-Shiff, 1993), displayed higher levels of anxiety than children outside the city. High schoolers from stricken neighborhoods expressed the greatest reservations about serving in the army in the near future (Israelshvili, 1992), and both elementary and high school pupils from such neighborhoods had the highest rates of general stress symptomatology and PTSD both a month and a year after the war's end (Schwarzwald et al., in press).

These findings are consistent with previous reports showing a high level of exposure to extreme stress to be a powerful risk factor for children (Milgram, Toubiana, Klingman, & Raviv, 1988; Pynoos & Eth, 1985). In particular, the finding that children whose homes had been hit suffered the greatest emotional damage (Schwarzwald et al., 1993) is consistent with findings of the study by Pynoos et al. (1987), cited above, of children whose school playground was attacked by snipers. That study found that the children who were actually in the playground at the time of the attacks showed more distress than those who were not at school or had left the school earlier in the day.

## Age

Although none of the studies made a comparative assessment of the stress responses of children of all ages, younger children were consistently shown to be more adversely affected than older ones by the Gulf War. Babies demonstrated more maladjustment than older toddlers (Rosenthal & Levy-Shiff, 1993); elementary school children showed more stress symtomatology and PTSD than junior high schoolers; and junior high schoolers demonstrated more stress than high schoolers (Klingman, 1992; Mintz, 1992; Raviv & Raviv, 1991; Schwarzwald et al., 1993).

Clinicians and researchers disagree widely as to whether older or younger children are the most vulnerable to disasters. As summarized by Gibbs (1989), Gleser et al. (1981), who compared children aged 2–20, found that the older the child, the more seriously he or she was affected by the Buffalo Creek flood. Eth and Pynoos (1985) reported that pre-school children are the most severely affected by serious trauma. Kins-ton and Rosser (1974) conclude from their literature review (which did not cover all age groups) that, of all children, 9- to 14-year-olds suffer the most emotional damage in disasters.

The findings of the Gulf War studies reported here are most consis-tent with those of Eth and Pynoos (1985) and similarly suggest that what makes younger children more vulnerable is their lack of cognitive and coping skills. According to Eth and Pynoos, adolescents have greater cognitive skills than their juniors; these skills enable them to formulate a greater variety of cognitive reappraisals and inner plans of action, which may allow for more flexible and efficient coping. Both the semi-projective study by Zeidner, et al. (1993) and the study by Weisenberg et al. (1993) on the relation between wartime coping and short-term post-war distress show an inverse relation between situationally effective cop-ing and anxiety. Though neither study adequately defines the overall type of coping that was most effective under the circumstances, there is some indication in the study by Weisenberg et al. that the ability of older children to distract themselves or to ignore the threat was of use. This is consistent with Rofe and Lewin's (1982) contention that young people living in stressful environments from which they cannot escape reduce their anxiety by shutting out the stressful material from conscious aware-ness.

The general thrust of the findings on the Gulf War would suggest that, of all children, infants and preschoolers are the most vulnerable to emotional damage in war and that, as a group, children suffer more distress than adults. However, the fact that none of the studies assessed all children's age groups, and the difficulty, also noted by Gibbs (1989), of comparing children's and adults' responses to disaster, rule out any definite assertion to this effect. Indeed, the inevitable differences in the measures used, stemming both from differences in the specific war ex-periences of the children and adults and from differences in the ways in which children and adults express distress, make it quite impossible to make quantitative comparisons of the Gulf War findings on the two pop-ulations. We have no measure that would indicate whether one or the other suffered more fear and anxiety, displayed more somatic symptoms, and so forth. The one study that assessed the level of fear among both children and adults found that children reported less fear than their mothers and more fear than their fathers (Rosenbaum & Ronen, 1992). But this does not tell what the pattern would be outside the family framework. More studies are clearly called for.

## Gender

Several of the studies found that girls reacted to the Gulf War with more stress than boys (Greenbaum et al., 1992; Klingman, in press; Mintz, 1992; Schwarzwald et al., 1993; Weisenberg et al., 1993). This is consistent with the finding of greater stress among adult women than men in the war (Chapter 4), but not consistent with previous literature. Milgram and Milgram (1976) reported that during the 1973 Yom Kippur War, boys' anxiety increased much more sharply than girls'. Burke et al. (1982) similarly found that first-grade boys showed stronger stress effects than the same-age girls after a blizzard, though a follow-up study (Burke, Moccia, Borus, & Burns, 1986) when the children were in the fifth grade showed that only the girls in this older sample still bore the distress of that event. More comprehensively, a research review by Zaslow and Hayes (1986) suggests that elementary school boys are more strongly affected than girls by single life events such as divorce and illness or death in the family. Recently, Hoffman, Levy-Shiff, Solberg, and Zarizki (1992) found that multiple life events were associated with increased anxiety and reduced assertiveness in a sample of fourth- through sixth-grade Israeli boys but not girls.

Neither the source of the gender difference in the Gulf War nor the source of the discrepancy with the literature is clear. Ronen and Rahav (1991), who found no gender differences in changes in children's stress-related habits during the Gulf War, suggest that the absence of such differences may have been due to the fact that their study measured behaviors rather than feelings. The gender differences found in the children's responses to the Gulf War may be explained by the same factors that were used to explain those found among adults, ranging from gender-biased measures and gender-based reporting of stress, on the one hand, through poorer coping skills and greater sensitivity to the suffering of others among females than males, on the other.

The effort to reach a large number of children in a very short time has led to the almost exclusive use of questionnaires in the studies of children's reactions to the Gulf War. Whether the questionnaires were answered by the children themselves or by their parents, they have clear limitations. Klingman et al. (1993), for example, point out that question-naires may not provide sufficient insight into the deeper level of psycho-logical functioning. Such contents might be better revealed by indirect methods such as examination of children's art or play and the use of clinical interviews, where feelings that might be repressed or denied at the conscious, verbal level could be better discerned. Nonetheless, the consistent pattern of findings observed across several studies, conducted independently by different groups of investigators, using a wide variety of instruments, lends validity to their common conclusions.

# 6

# Holocaust Survivors
# in the Gulf War

## THE GULF WAR AS A STRESSOR FOR THE AGED

The Gulf War posed particular stresses for Israel's elderly, who make up over 10% of the country's population.

As in other wars, essential social services were kept running, but many "nonessential" ones were radically curtailed. Thus the senior citizens' centers to which many elderly came for everything from company to instrumental services were shut down in the afternoons and evenings. In a war in which people in general tended to stay indoors, the elderly were more housebound than usual and thus more isolated.

The emergency procedures also posed special problems for the elderly. Many of them lacked the manual dexterity needed to fit the gas masks and had even more difficulty than their juniors in getting themselves settled in the sealed room in the short time allotted. Some coped by sealing up their entire apartment, which meant that they spent long hours in sunless, airless confinement. For those with impaired vision or hearing, seclusion in the sealed room often aggravated their sense of isolation. Some had trouble hearing the air-raid sirens; yet others found it difficult to understand the emergency instructions broadcast over the radio and television.

To make matters worse, the elderly had the misfortune of being concentrated in the high-risk greater Tel Aviv area, where they made up 14% of the population (Central Bureau of Statistics, 1992). While many younger people left for safer terrain, the elderly tended to stay put, lacking the means, energy, and perhaps incentive to leave.

The first question that this chapter asks is how these people fared during the war.

## COPING DIFFICULTIES OF THE AGED

The best answer we have to this question is provided by the survey, discussed in Chapter 2, carried out by the Israel Defense Forces' (IDF) Department of Behavioral Sciences. Among those surveyed were a representative sample of Israel's aged. The findings were that while the aged were similar to their juniors in attitudes and behavior, they had a harder time coping.

The study found that the elderly did not differ significantly from the rest of the population in their knowledge of the protective procedures, their satisfaction with the amount and clarity of the media information on the subject, and their performance of the emergency instructions. That is, about the same proportion of elderly obeyed instructions to seal rooms and wear gas masks as the rest, and about the same proportions did and did not hoard food and supplies. As the authors of the study explain it, Israel's elderly are well versed in wars and did not need a great deal of prompting to do what was required under the circumstances.

Similarly, there were no significant differences in the faith that the two populations had in the army high command or in their agreement with the policy of restraint, which were high in both groups. Nor were there significant differences in their faith in the protective devices and procedures, which was low.

The aged did, however, differ from the rest of the adult population in two ways. One is that they found the war less disruptive of their daily routine and work and less damaging economically than did their juniors. This difference is self-evident.

More telling is that throughout most of the war they felt that they managed less well. Figure 6.1 shows the coping reported by the two populations at various points of the war. As can be seen, at the start of the war, the aged coped only slightly less well (the difference was not statistically significant) than the rest of the population. With the Ramat Gan missile strikes, however, their sense of mastery plummeted. While the rest of the population reported that they coped better as the war progressed, throughout much of that period the aged reported that they coped worse. It was only toward the very end of the war, when the missile strikes were few and far between and tended to be off target, that their coping improved and reached the level of that of the rest of the population.

In other words, the study suggests that while on a practical level the

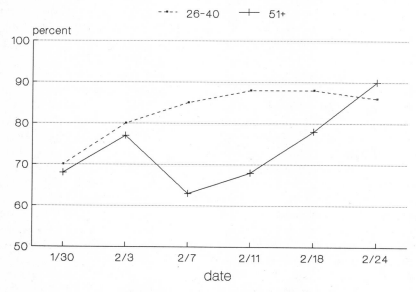

**Figure 6.1.** Coping over time by age.

aged apparently continued to function during the war, obeying the emergency instructions and going on with their lives, emotionally they found it harder than their juniors to cope with the destructive missile strikes, and they suffered greater and longer-lasting distress in their wake.

This is the only formal study of the aged available at this point, but impressionistic testimony consistent with its findings are provided in an unpublished paper by a social worker, Ada Barzilai, who worked with a group of residents of an old-age home in Tel Aviv. The residents in the home were 80 years of age of older. Barzilai's report (unpublished manuscript) tells of adaptive coping behavior by most of the residents along with a great deal of tension and anxiety. On the one hand, they tended to view the situation realistically and kept themselves informed by watching television, listening to the radio, attending the daily news summaries she gave, asking the staff about events, and discussing the situation with one another. Barzilai observes that there was a thirst for information not typical of peacetime and an even more atypical cessation of interpersonal conflicts and competition for status and staff attention. She also noticed many examples of mutual help, thoughtfulness, and new friendships. On the other hand, the anxiety of the elderly residents was palpable, manifesting itself in irritability, oversensitivity to noise, and sleep disturbances.

These findings are consistent with those of an earlier study by Hobfoll, Lomranz, Eyal, Bridges, and Tzemach (1989) that showed that aged

Israelis in the Lebanon War reacted to that war with extremely high levels of depression. They differ, however, from the findings of several studies that indicate that the elderly cope better with stress than do younger people. Bell (1978) demonstrated that the elderly cope better than younger people with both natural disasters and disasters caused by human beings. Bolin and Klenow (1982–1983) found that older persons are less adversely affected by disasters than their juniors. Melick and Logue (1985–1986) found that the elderly are not seriously affected by extreme stress at all. These authors suggest that having experienced such stressful life events as war, death, divorce, and bereavement, the aged develop the ability and resources to cope with extreme stress.

Several reasons can be suggested as to why age did not confer a similar advantage to the Israeli elderly in the Gulf War.

One, as already noted, is that the Gulf War may have been more stressful for the aged than for younger people. In particular, the war exacerbated the loneliness in which many elderly people live. Not only were the activities of the community centers where many of them go for company curtailed, but social life in general was radically reduced during the war. People avoided unnecessary excursions. Come evening, Scud time, they immured themselves in their four walls. During daylight hours, they visited less, shopped less, and spent less time in parks and cafés and on the streets than Israelis, taking advantage of the country's Mediterranean climate, ordinarily do. This constriction had double implications for the elderly. It is likely that however few friends and relatives may have visited them before the war, fewer came calling now and called less often. At the same time, the elderly probably stayed home more than most, not being forced out and into contact with others by jobs, by public obligations like school duty, or by the need to shop and do errands for their families, as younger people were. Since many elderly live alone, it is quite conceivable that they spent days on end without human company.

Another reason the aged did not cope better than younger people may have to do with the nature of the life experience Israel's elderly have accrued. The studies cited above deal mostly with life experiences that can be expected in the natural course of events. Few people reach a ripe old age without having had family problems, lost someone close to them, been ill, or suffered some other personal tragedy. But the life experience of most elderly Israelis includes not only these personal crises but also major disasters.

Few if any elderly Israelis have not been subjected to some major catastrophe or displacement. Most are immigrants who came to Israel from very different societies and have had to make substantial adjustments in their way of life. Many were refugees who either fled their home countries or sneaked out surreptitiously, braving many dangers to reach Israel and leaving most of their possessions behind. Many had suffered persecution or pogroms in the period before their immigration.

Moreover, both they and the "old-timers" who had arrived earlier in the century, before the creation of the State and out of volition rather than compulsion, lived through numerous wars punctuated by uneasy, uncertain periods not of peace but of short-lived nonbelligerency (Milgram, 1978). Even these periods were punctuated by terrorist attacks, border incursions, and, in recent years, the Intifada. Israel has more than its share of war widows and of parents who have lived to see their sons killed in combat. The experience of war is woven relentlessly through the family and professional lives of most elderly Israelis.

Something of the flavor of the Israeli experience of war is conveyed by the life of Ra'anan Weitz, who was born in 1913 in Rehovot, one of modern Israel's first Jewish settlements. Weitz's earliest memories begin with war: the recollection of Turkish soldiers begging his father for bread as they escaped the British army entering Palestine in 1917. In high school, Weitz already had his first military experience, when, in 1929, the year of Arab attacks on the Jews of Hebron and Mozah, he and other students volunteered to stand guard over a village in the Jerusalem area. He remembers himself and four other boys listening petrified to the cries ringing through the air on the night of the Mozah Massacre. In 1936, a student of agriculture, he went to the Galilee to help defend Jewish settlements there against attack by neighboring Arabs. During World War II, with a wife and a doctorate in agriculture in hand, he volunteered to serve in the Jewish Brigade of the British army and was sent to Europe. After the war, he took part in clandestine operations to bring Jewish Holocaust survivors to Israel in defiance of British immigration restrictions. He fought in the 1948 War of Independence, during which his brother was killed, then in the 1956 Sinai Campaign. In the Six Day War of 1967 he was still on active duty. By the Yom Kippur War of 1973 he was too old to fight, but was sent to assess the damage caused by the Syrian attack on the Golan Heights settlements. In his seventies, he sat out the 1982 Lebanon War and the subsequent Intifada, but, like other Israelis, he could not help but be a close witness.

Ra'anan Weitz is something of a mythical figure in Israel's history, a kind of Renaissance soldier-scholar-statesman, with a worldwide reputation as an agronomist and an illustrious political career at home, where he was active in pre-State settlement and subsequent nation building. These enlarged proportions notwithstanding, the dense interweave of wars in his family and professional life is typical of Israel's aged. If not all of Israelis elderly lived through as many wars as Weitz, one would be hard put to find a pensioner who had seen no wars. And if they did not all don uniforms and fight, as the women did not, then they were repeatedly exposed to the anxiety of having sons, other relatives, and friends on the front and the grief of losing loved ones and acquaintances in battle. Moreover, they were themselves part of a population whose lives were continually threatened to some degree or another.

What all this translates into is that the bulk of Israel's elderly population has lived though situations (emphatically plural) that at best were enormously stressful and at worst potentially pathogenic. The many wars they endured are of a very different order of stressor than the life events that may make for resilience to stress and for equanimity in crisis.

The third possible reason for the greater vulnerability of the aged in this study has to do with the nature of the stressor: a war. The Gulf War was yet another war in the lives of people who were heartily weary of war. A study that I conducted with my colleagues in the army (Solomon, Mikulincer, & Jacob, 1987) has found that after a soldier's second war, every war he fights makes him more susceptible to a psychiatric breakdown in battle. It seems that the overexposure of Israel's aged to war has also made them vulnerable to the stresses of war.

## AGED HOLOCAUST SURVIVORS: DISCOMFORTING ASSOCIATIONS

The remainder of this chapter turns to one particular segment of Israel's elderly population: survivors of the Nazi Holocaust. Holocaust survivors constitute about half of the population age 60 and over in Israel (Amcha, 1991). In addition to the stresses that the war created for the rest of the elderly population, Holocaust survivors experienced special stresses of their own.

Certain features of the Gulf War bore a disturbing resemblance to aspects of the Holocaust. These included the often repeated threat of gas, the machinations of a megalomaniacal tyrant, and the targeting of unarmed civilians. As the journalist Anat Meidan (1991), daughter of survivors, tells it, "When you sit in that room, with your mother and father who survived the Warsaw Ghetto, you cannot escape from the amazing resemblance: people who survived the gas chambers of Auschwitz are now pressing themselves into a gas mask that will hopefully save them from the same German gas."

Furthermore, the prominent Israeli psychologist Shlomo Breznitz, himself a child survivor of the Holocaust, points out the Iraqis have used the Holocaust to instill fear. In his autobiographic book Breznitz wrote:

As I dwell on the fate of my family during those darkest of days in Europe, Baghdad Radio is boasting that Iraqi Scud missiles have turned Tel Aviv into a "crematorium." That was their exact word, aired today, January 19, 1991. They could have phrased it differently, using any of a number of alternatives: devastation, misery, defeat, desert, wasteland, destruction, ruin, fall, havoc or even fire or hell. But the word they chose, taken from the unholy vocabulary that dominated my childhood, was targeted to hit the most vulnerable part of their victims' souls, with a precision, exceeding by far that of the missiles themselves. It did not start today, for some time already Saddam Hussein has been threatening the newly gathered survivors of the Holocaust with chemical annihilation. Touché! This man must know some history— at least in the crudest, most rudimentary sense. (1992, p. 65)

For many of the survivors, the associations brought disturbing memories. As Meidan (1991) tells, "The Gulf War brought up out of the basement memories of days gone by. Horror stories, long re-pressed, float into the space of the sealed room." The psychiatrist Dr. Arik Shalev of Haddassah Hopsital in Jerusalem provides an especially vivid example in his account of an agitated 60-year-old orthopedic pa-tient whom he was called in to see on the night of the first alarm. As Dr. Shalev reports, "This good man said that he could see piles of dead bodies every time he closed his eyes, the same bodies that he had actu-ally seen in the concentration camp. He was used to having nightmares and was not afraid of them nor of being confined to bed during the alarm. But he wanted to talk because he no longer wished to live. 'It's back again,' he said, 'the gas, the hatred. It wasn't worth trying a new life'" (Shalev, 1991a).

The Israeli media picked up on the associations. In the press, and on radio and television, Saddam was compared to Hitler, his rise to Hitler's rise, his German-made bunker to Hitler's bunker, the reportedly German-made gas he threatened Israel with to the gas used in the death camps. Almost every day, Holocaust survivors were interviewed, and their views and experiences were printed and broadcast.

The media gave expression to a wide range of views. Many of the survivors cited were evidently profoundly disturbed by the associations between the Holocaust and the Gulf War. One example is found in a support group run by the Israeli organization Amcha (National Israeli Center for Psychological Support of Survivors of the Holocaust and the Second Generation), where we hear such statements as the following:

What I feel is that all my life they want to destroy the Jews. Now I feel bad because again we have to sit back quietly and not react.

I feel degraded by the thought that others are fighting for us. I came here after Auschwitz. Three weeks after I arrived at the kibbutz I was holding a gun in my hand. Now, this passivity takes me back 45 years. During this time I detached myself from the Holocaust. I didn't read, didn't see films, never told my children, but, oddly, this war awakened the same feelings of degradation I felt in Auschwitz. (Galili, 1991)

Other survivors hotly denied any similarities and disclaimed fear. For example, the poet Helena Birenbaum claimed to have put the past firmly behind her:

> My motto is: the past is gone, the present is what counts. Whatever happened before, whether yesterday or forty years ago, has been erased. Today, when I put the mask on my face, I don't think of Zyklon B [the gas used in the extermination camps]; I think only of Saddam's missiles. The Holocaust is far away. It's over. I came out of it. Let's say I'd had an operation and then twenty years later had to have the same surgery again—would I think about the first operation or about what was happening now? Of course I'd think only about what was awaiting me without relating it to the past. Today I live in another reality, in another country. I have children and grandchildren. My fears are different. (Meidan, 1991)

Similarly, Miriam Zeiger, chairperson of the Mengele Twins Organization, asserted:

> As someone whose whole family was annihilated in Auschwitz in the gas chambers, I am not afraid, and I hardly ever use the mask. (Meidan, 1991)

If these disavowals seem a bit rigid and perhaps intimate a certain lack of resolution of the Holocaust trauma, they also give voice to the recognition by many survivors of the vast difference in the destructiveness and hardships of the two events and to their realization that their position during the Gulf War—living in their own country, with adequate food and shelter, surrounded by family and friends, and backed up by the Israel's strong army that, though momentarily inactive, could, if needed, defend them—was infinitely better than what it had been in the Holocaust.

Whatever the views presented, the media struck a resonant chord. Its intense occupation with the Holocaust in the weeks leading up to the Gulf War and all the while that the war was being fought expressed a general sense that the Holocaust was a legitimate and meaningful point of reference, both for the survivors and for the Israelis who read or heard what they had to say. But beyond that, it also reflected the intuition on the part of nonprofessionals that people who had survived the Holocaust would respond to the Gulf War from the vantage point of that ordeal.

## HOW THE STUDY CAME ABOUT

The idea for this study came to me when I was sitting with my mother, a survivor of Auschwitz, in the sealed room. The last war in which my mother and I had been together was the 1967 Six Day War, almost a quarter of a century earlier. I was in adolescence, she in middle age, a healthy, well-organized, and supportive woman who served as an anchor in the tense weeks before Israel's preemptive strike and during the short week of fighting. While my sister and I were gripped by the fear prevalent throughout the Israeli population that the country would be annihilated, my mother seemed a pillar of strength and a model of calm.

In the Gulf War, she was a different woman altogether. When the alarm sounded, she retreated into a corner of the sealed room and seemed to curl up into herself, practically oblivious to the radio, to her two grandchildren, and to my husband and myself. She fumbled with her mask, and on a number of occasions she would certainly have choked had one of us not removed the protective cap that sealed the filter when the mask was not in use.

In part, her behavior could be attributed to age, infirmity, and grief. She was 69 years old, ill, and in mourning for my father who had died two years earlier. But I felt that there was more involved than her strictly personal circumstances. For from her corner, from way inside herself, she kept repeating, "I can't any more. I've had enough wars." It seemed to me that ultimately it was her experience in Auschwitz that was behind her "giving in and giving up" in the Gulf War, and I wondered how other Holocaust survivors responded. Was my mother's intense distress idiosyncratic, or did other Holocaust survivors share it? Since I coped with my war-related anxieties by keeping busy with my work, I decided to research the question.

It was not immediately clear how this could be done in wartime and without any official list of Holocaust survivors from which to obtain a sample population. I was helped in this quandary by Dr. Shimon Spiro, dean of the Tel Aviv University School of Social Work, who introduced me to Dr. Edward Prager. Prager was in charge of gerontology studies. He opened many doors for me, and we collaborated on a study.

## HOLOCAUST SURVIVORS

The professional literature on Holocaust survivors strongly suggests that they are a vulnerable population,. Beginning in the 1960s, a considerable body of both clinical (for example, Choddof, 1986; Dasberg, 1987; Eitinger, 1965, 1980; Krystal, 1981) and research (for example, Danieli, 1981) literature has pointed to serious long-term emotional disturbances among Holocaust survivors. Neiderland (1968) and Eitinger (1965) identified a complex of symptoms, including emotional detachment and constriction, chronic depression, anxiety, fear of the future, memory impairment, trouble concentrating, and recurrent nightmares of the trauma, which are today recognized as part of the posttraumatic stress syndrome that may afflict victims of any catastrophe, whether natural or caused by human beings (APA, 1987). Other findings are that concentration camp survivors are more pessimistic than comparable controls (Lomranz, Shmotkin, Zchovoi, & Rosenberg, 1985; Shuval, 1963); display less sense of well-being, lower emotional health, and less role satisfaction (Antonovsky, Maoz, Dowty, & Wijsenbeek, 1971); and show more cognitive and personality constriction (Dor-Shav, 1978; Shanan & Shahar, 1983). The damage has been seen as so profound that it affected not only the survivors themselves but also the emotional constellations of their children (Barocas & Barocas, 1979; Bergmann & Jacovy, 1982; Danieli, 1980; Epstein, 1983).

In recent years, there has also been literature of the special difficulties that aged survivors face. Nadler (1983) points out that in old age, when the tasks of rebuilding a life and family are over and the survivors' attention is no longer centered on practical tasks in the external world, the psychological effects of traumatization resurface. Lomranz (1990) similarly suggests that the posttraumatic responses that the survivors controlled and subordinated to the tasks of day-to-day living while they were in early and middle adulthood may be reactivated in old age. Dasberg (1987) holds that the "late effects" of Holocaust traumatization "increase, rather than abate with advancing age" (p. 250).

On the other hand, various authors have argued that the survivors are on the whole an emotionally healthy group. Leon, Butcher, Kleinman, Goldberg, and Almagor (1981) argue that only a minority of the survivors suffer the serious consequences pointed to in these studies and that most live productive lives without major psychological impairment. Yet others recognize the vulnerabilities of survivors but contend that they cope better with hardship than do comparable controls. Shuval (1963) found that concentration camp survivors faced the difficulties of the immigrant camps in Israel with less increase in pessimism than European nonsurvivors. Shanan & Shahar (1983) found that in crises Holocaust survivors used more active coping strategies than did controls.

## THE EFFECT OF PRIOR TRAUMA: VULNERABILITY OR RESILIENCE?

Although there is a great deal of evidence to the effect that Holocaust survivors, and especially aged Holocaust survivors, are a vulnerable group, the literature still leaves open the question of how they would cope with stress in general and with stress reminiscent of their

Holocaust ordeal in particular. Does their Holocaust experience impair their coping? Or, might it make them better equipped to deal with hardship?

The literature on coping offers two contradictory views: the inoculation perspective and the vulnerability perspective.

## The Inoculation Perspective

The inoculation perspective holds that stress contributes to the development of useful coping strategies: that each similar hardship increases familiarity, leading to a decrease in the amount of perceived stress and enabling more successful adaptation in future stressful situations (Epstein, 1983; Janis, 1971; Keinan, 1979). Eysenck (1983) refines this view somewhat by proposing the utility of both similar and dissimilar stressors. A stressor, he states, can promote either "direct tolerance" of *similar* stressors in the future and/or "indirect tolerance" of *dissimilar* stressors.

A study by Norris and Murrel (1988) on elderly flood victims in a flood-prone region of Appalachia is particularly relevant to the question at hand. Norris and Murrel found that elderly flood victims who had lived through a flood earlier in their lives endured a subsequent one with less anxiety and weather-related distress than their age mates who had not had that prior experience. Norris and Murrel's findings support the utility of similar stressors. The studies cited above that found that the aged in general fared better than younger people in crisis provide support for the utility of dissimilar stressors.

Applied to Holocaust survivors, the inoculation perspective would expect that they weathered the Gulf War with either greater equanimity than their age mates, if the direct tolerance model is advanced, or with the same equanimity, if the cross-tolerance model is the basis for prediction.

## The Vulnerability Perspective

The vulnerability perspective considers repeated exposure to stressful events a risk factor. It holds that every stressful life event depletes available coping resources and thereby increases vulnerability to subsequent stress (Coleman, Butcher, & Carson, 1980; McGrath, 1970; Selye, 1956; Vinokur & Selzer, 1975).

Numerous studies of posttrauma point to the pathogenic affect of recurrent exposure. Silver and Wortman (1980) found that people who had experienced extreme stress in the past were more vulnerable to the aftereffects of subsequent stressors. Similarly, Solomon, Mikulincer, and Jacob (1987) found that the accumulated stress of multiple wars had a largely detrimental impact on the ability of soldiers to retain their emotional equilibrium in battle. Soldiers who had stress reactions in their first war were more likely to break down in the second, while soldiers who weathered their first war emotionally intact became candidates for breakdowns by the time they faced their second. Other studies suggest that exposure to traumatic events leaves the victims more vulnerable in general. Solomon, Oppenheimer, Elizur, and Waysman (1990) found that after a soldier was traumatized in war, he did not return to his prewar level of control—even after he coped successfully with a subsequent war. Titchner (1986; Titchner & Ross, 1974) has argued strongly that exposure to a traumatic event may issue in a process of posttraumatic decline and leave permanent characterological effects, especially proneness to anxiety reactions.

Applied to Holocaust survivors, the vulnerability perspective would predict that they fared much worse than other elderly during the Gulf War, whether that war is regarded as a similar stressor or merely a symbolic reminder of the first.

## THE STUDY OF HOLOCAUST SURVIVORS IN THE GULF WAR

The present study addressed the question of whether Holocaust survivors responded differently to the Gulf War than their non-Holocaust age mates and, if so, how. Did they respond with more anxiety or less? Or was there no substantial difference? To put it differently, did the trials they endured during the Holocaust help them cope with the difficulties of the Gulf War or evoke old anxieties that impaired their ability to manage?

To answer this question, we surveyed 192 senior citizens during the Gulf War. Sixty-one (31.8%) of the sample were Holocaust survivors; 131 (68.2%) were not. In the Holocaust group, the average age was 68.3, and 33.3% were male; in the non-Holocaust group, the average age was 72.9, and 38.5% were male. Twelve percent were residents of an urban community home for the aged; the rest all lived in their own homes.

Subjects were first presented with a brief questionnaire inquiring about sociodemographic variables: age, sex, education, religious observance, marital status, place of residence, country of origin, and current health status. They were then asked about the nature of their Holocaust experience, namely, whether they had been in concentration camps, in hiding, or with partisan bands.

This was followed by three sets of questions on other experiences that may have interacted with their Holocaust backgrounds in their response to the Gulf War. The first two assessed "objective" experiences. One dealt with other traumatic events—namely whether they had participated in other wars and whether they had lost family members in war. The other dealt with the personal life events (such as marriage, divorces, change of residence, illness, loss of employment) they had experienced. The third tried to assess the subjects' "subjective" experience and asked them to indicate whether they had ever experienced any event similar to the Gulf War in the past.

After these questions were completed, the subjects were presented with four questionnaires that measured (1) sense of danger, (2) self-efficacy, (3) war-related distress, and (4) state and trait anxiety (Spielberger, Gorsuch, & Lushene, 1970).

## FINDINGS

### War-Related and General Distress

The findings show that Holocaust survivors responded to the Gulf War with greater distress than elderly nonsurvivors (see Table 6.1). They viewed the war as more dangerous, rating their own danger, the danger of Israel's being annihilated, and the danger of the war to their families higher than did their nonsurvivor age mates. They displayed both greater state anxiety and greater trait anxiety than nonsurvivors, and significantly more survivors than nonsurvivors reported specifically war-

Table 6.1. Psychological Ratings during the Gulf War for Elderly Israeli Survivors of the Holocaust and Other Elderly Subjects[a]

| Measure | Holocaust survivors (N = 61) | | Other subjects (N = 131) | | F (df = 1,100) |
|---|---|---|---|---|---|
| | Mean | SD | Mean | SD | |
| Perceptions of danger | −0.2 | 0.9 | 0.5 | 1.1 | 2.29 |
| Psychological distress | 42.9 | 11.9 | 33.0 | 10.1 | 6.20 |
| State anxiety | 47.4 | 13.2 | 36.5 | 13.0 | 6.27 |
| Trait anxiety | 50.3 | 10.4 | 41.5 | 7.4 | 7.53[b] |

[a]A multivariate analysis of covariance was performed with age, sex, education, religiosity, health, and proximity to bomb sites as covariates. Overall $F = 2.43$, $df = 4, 97$, $p < 0.05$.
[b]$p < .005$, with Bonferroni correction. See Miller, 1981, for multiple comparisons.

related distress, in the form of sleep disturbances (68.9% versus 51.5%); concentration difficulties or memory impairment (54.1% versus 36.6%); apprehension and tension (80.3% versus 64%); nightmares (41% versus 23.7%); loss of interest in significant activities (59% versus 40.8%); sense of detachment from others (28.8% versus 10.4%); as well as stronger feelings of panic and fear (37.7% versus 16.9%, irritability (72% versus 46.2%), excitability (65.6% versus 48.1%), and hopelessness (42.6% versus 11.6%). In short, on four of the measures Holocaust survivors showed greater vulnerability than nonsurvivors. Moreover, with the exception of the sense of danger, the differences remained significant when the background factors that might bias the findings, including the differences in mean age and gender in the two groups, were controlled for.

## Impact of Other Life Experiences

The impact of other life experiences on the response of the subjects was assessed by a secondary analysis of the data set by Shira Hantman (1992) in her thesis for an MSW at the Tel Aviv University School of

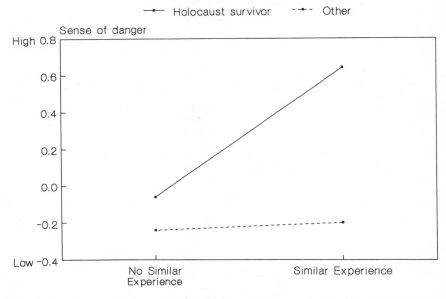

**Figure 6.2.** Interactive effects of the Holocaust, prior traumatic experiences, and sense of danger.

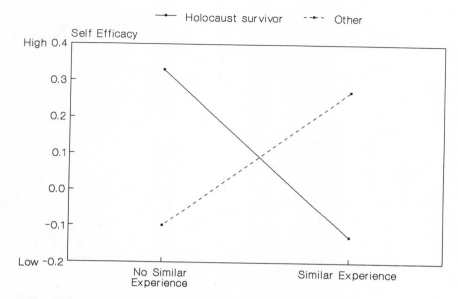

**Figure 6.3.** Interactive effects of the Holocaust, prior traumatic experiences, and self-efficacy.

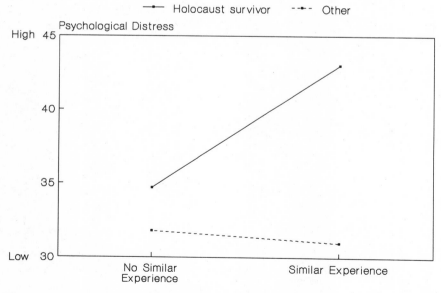

**Figure 6.4.** Interactive effects of the Holocaust, prior traumatic experiences, and level of distress.

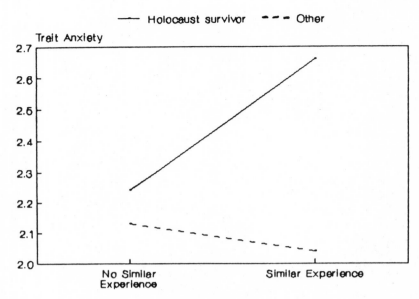

**Figure 6.5.** Interactive effects of the Holocaust, prior traumatic experiences, and trait anxiety.

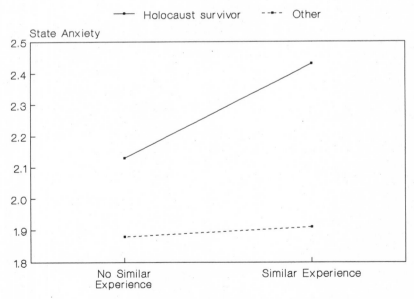

**Figure 6.6.** Interactive effects of the Holocaust, prior traumatic experiences, and state anxiety.

Social Work. This analysis focused on the effect of other prior traumatic experiences similar to those of the Gulf War.

The findings were oddly mixed. Surprisingly, none of the "objective" life events had any impact on how either the survivor or nonsurvivor group coped. On the other hand, the subjective sense of having experienced something like the Gulf War in the past had a significant impact on the coping of the survivors but not on that of the nonsurvivors.

As can be seen from Figures 6.2–6.6, Holocaust survivors who reported having had a prior experience similar to the Gulf War were even more vulnerable than other survivors. They reported feeling a significantly greater sense of danger, lower self-efficacy, and higher levels of trait, though not of state, anxiety. Among non-Holocaust survivors, no such differences were found. Neither their sense of danger, self-efficacy, nor anxiety were affected by whether or not they had a prior experience similar to the Gulf War.

## VULNERABILITY IN A NONCLINICAL POPULATION

The findings clearly show that Holocaust survivors were more vulnerable during the Gulf War than nonsurivors. In this, the findings are consistent with the abundance of other studies that point to the pervasive, long-lasting damage of exposure to traumatic events.

Unlike most studies of Holocaust survivors, the current study was based on a nonclinical sample. Its findings that the Holocaust survivors surveyed during the Gulf War showed greater acute distress and sense of danger, lower self-efficacy, and higher levels of both state and trait anxiety than a control group of the same ethnic and cultural background indicate the pervasive detrimental impact of the Holocaust. The findings show that psychological difficulties affected not only help-seeking survivors (those who *admit* to psychological problems) but also many survivors who tried to rebuild their lives by putting the Holocaust behind them.

The various findings to the effect that survivors coped less well during the Gulf War than their non-Holocaust age mates, displaying greater sense of danger, higher state and trait anxiety, and more symptoms of war-related stress, are indicative of the residue of stress left by the Holocaust in the survivors' lives. Together these findings show that the survivors retain from their Holocaust experience both a generalized sensitivity to stress and a more specific sensitivity to the stress of war. In this, the findings are consistent with the evidence cited above to the effect that survivors suffer from psychological difficulties that can be traced back to their Holocaust ordeal (for example, Eitinger, 1980;

Neiderland, 1968). They are also consistent with the findings that the survivors are particularly susceptible to the resurgence of Holocaust-related memories, anxieties, and stresses in old age (Dasberg, 1987; Lomranz, 1990; Nadler, 1989).

Although they do not show it directly, the findings do suggest that for many survivors the Gulf War exacerbated or reactivated the trauma of the Holocaust. Evidence of the reactivation of earlier war-related trauma during the aging process has been provided by a number of researchers. In a 20-year follow-up of American veterans, Archibald and Tuddenham (1965) found that symptoms of traumatic stress that had been latent since their war experience became evident during the aging process. Christenson, Walker, Ross, and Maltbie (1981) report experiences consistent with these findings. Over the years they found increasing numbers of World War II veterans who "showed exacerbation of symptoms of a traumatic stress disorder." Presenting a case of a reactivation "precipitated by an event that simulated the original trauma," they went on to suggest that "losses associated with involutional age, including parental loss, children leaving home, pending retirement and increasing medical disability all serve as stressors that may reactivate a latent traumatic stress disorder" (p. 985).

Moreover, studies of reactivation of traumas in the civilian sphere have shown that reactivation can occur after many years of dormancy and can be triggered by events only remotely reminiscent of the original trauma. For example, it has been shown that reactivation of unresolved grief reactions, in which the bereaved are suddenly reemerged in the mourning process, with all its attendant feelings of sadness, pining, and depression, can be triggered by a large range of events from deliberate recall through incidental reminders of the death (Lindeman, 1944). Similarly, among rape victims, Burgess and Halmstrom (1974) and Notman and Nadelson (1976) report unresolved feelings emerging many years after the assault, giving rise to acute depression, anxiety, and phobic behaviors much like those commonly experienced in the period immediately following a rape. These findings on the reactivation of bereavement and rape reactions suggest that it was indeed the association of the Gulf War with the Holocaust, however remote the actual resemblance may have been, and the power of that association to exacerbate or trigger reactivations of the survivors' Holocaust trauma, that made the war such a potent stressor.

In the context of the above studies of reactivation, we can suggest that the Holocaust survivors proved so vulnerable during the Gulf War because the interplay of the susceptibility of age joined with the evocative power of the Gulf War. This interplay may explain the discrepancy between the current findings and the findings cited above that Holocaust survivors dealt better with hardships than comparable nonsurvivors (Shanan & Shahar, 1983; Shuval, 1963). The studies that reached that optimistic conclusion were conducted when the survivors were younger as a group and considered stressors that bore less resemblance to the Holocaust than did the Gulf War.

The current findings are also quite the reverse of Norris and Murrel's (1988) finding, noted above, that elderly flood victims who had experienced prior floods fared emotionally better than those who had not. The Holocaust experience of the elderly survivors in our study did not similarly help them cope with the Gulf War. The discrepancy may be accounted for by two reasons.

One is that Israel's Holocaust survivors are part of the same aged population discussed above that has experienced more potentially traumatic hardship than elderly people in less war-ridden parts of the world. As a subgroup within that population, Israel's Holocaust survivors experienced even more traumatic events. Our findings suggest that even if life's "ordinary" stressors and natural disasters may strengthen a person's ability to cope, a massive catastrophe like the Holocaust by and large depletes it.

The other, not unrelated, explanation is that disasters caused by humans wreak a great deal more emotional damage than natural ones (Beigel & Berren, 1985; Fields, 1980; Fredrick, 1980; Navon, 1992). Navon (1992) attributes the difference to the tendency of people to perceive the victims of human violence, as opposed to the victims of natural catastrophes, as at least partly responsible for their plight and to the aspersion that entails. This explanation would be supported by the cool reception that Holocaust survivors received when they first arrived in Israel, when they were blamed for everything from going to their deaths like sheep to the slaughter to using unscrupulous means to survive.

At the same time, it has been frequently pointed out that traumatic events undermine the victims' basic trust and their belief in the goodness and continuity of the world (Janoff-Bullman, 1989). It might be argued that since survivors of human-made disasters experience not only the unreliability of nature but also the cruelty and treachery of people, the damage to their trust is that much more extensive.

## INTENSIFICATION OF STRESS
## THROUGH OTHER EXPERIENCES

The "prior events" queried in this study were of two kinds: specific "objective" events ranging from the traumatic (for example, participation in combat, death of a family member in war) to ordinary life events, and "subjective" events reminiscent of the Gulf War. Unlike the two questions about previous traumatic and life experiences, the question "Have you ever experienced an event similar to the Gulf War before?" is open-ended and nonspecific. Subjects who answered in the affirmative were not asked to indicate or describe the event. It could have been any of Israel's wars, the Holocaust, or anything else that came to mind. The purpose of the question was to tap the respondents' subjective perception of the Gulf War—that is, whether or not the Gulf War evoked associations with other events in their lives. As pointed out earlier, some Holocaust survivors linked the Gulf War with the Holocaust, whereas others denied any similarity. The question attempted to differentiate between individuals for whom the Gulf War was simply another war whose stresses could be dealt with as they came and those for whom it echoed and reverberated with other stressful experiences—whatever they may have been. The analysis then attempted to discern what impact those reverbations had on both the aged Holocaust survivors and the aged non-Holocaust survivors in Israel.

The finding that the sense of a previous similar experience did not affect the response of the nonsurvivors to the war while it amplified the distress of the survivors is yet additional evidence of the survivors' greater vulnerability.

The finding that survivors who reported having had an earlier experience similar to the Gulf War showed more distress than those who did not points to the ability of a similar earlier stressor—even if that similarity is purely subjective—both to reactivate and intensify the later stress it resembles. The finding is consistent with the findings of a series of studies conducted on Israeli soldiers in the Lebanon War who had sustained traumatic or posttraumatic reactions in previous conflicts (Solomon, 1993). These studies found that the more reminiscent the soldier's Lebanon encounter was of his earlier traumatic experience, the more likely it was to exacerbate residual symptoms or to trigger a reactivation of his previous stress reaction. Like the Gulf War, the later stressor did not have to be as intense as the first or even of objectively major dimensions; it was enough that in the soldier's mind it resembled the first and evoked memories and associations.

The finding can also be explained by the cumulative impact of trauma. According to the Israeli clinical psychologist Emanuel Berman (1985), a second trauma neither heals an earlier trauma nor provides an opportunity for correction. Berman argues that trauma deepens trauma: that each traumatic event intensifies the threat inherent in the next one and augments the victim's vulnerability and distress.

The finding that none of the objective stresses queried—neither participation in other wars, the loss of loved ones, nor any stressful life event—affected the survivors' coping with the Gulf War brings home the importance of the subjective meaning of an event in the reactivation of earlier traumas. Although it is common to speak of the survivors as a group, individual survivors undoubtedly differ in how well they worked through their experience. Their subjective feelings during and about the Gulf War may be one index of that working-through. This interpretation suggests that the survivors who sustained the most serious and long-lasting psychological injuries in the Holocaust were the ones who reported both previous experiences similar to the Gulf War and the strongest distress during the war.

## TRAIT ANXIETY

While most of the measures in this study assess the specific impact of the Holocaust on the survivors' coping in the Gulf War, the trait anxiety measure taps the more pervasive and general residue of the trauma. As we recall, the Holocaust survivors displayed significantly higher trait anxiety than nonsurvivors. However, the trait anxiety of the nonsurvivors seems to be inordinately high as well.

Returning to Table 6.1, we see that the average trait anxiety score for Holocaust survivors was 50.3, and for non-Holocaust survivors it was 41.5. While to our knowledge there are no comparable studies of the aged in wartime with which to compare our findings, we can get a sense of the severity of their anxiety by viewing the scores against norms suggested by Himmelfarb and Murrel (1983, 1984) in two large-scale studies of the aged in a community in Kentucky. On the basis of their study, which compared a group of elderly people in a community sample in Kentucky with a group of elderly psychiatric inpatients, these authors determined that a trait anxiety score of 44 on the Speilberger inventory distinguished between them; and they subsequently used this cutoff point to identify individuals "at risk for a degree of psychological distress that would require intervention" (Himmelfarb & Murrel, 1984, p. 162). The Holocaust survivors in the current study scored considerably higher than this demarcation point, and the non-Holocaust aged did not score all that much lower.

The mean anxiety score for our sample—43.84—when the scores of survivors and nonsurvivors are averaged, is also considerably higher than the mean trait anxiety score of 33.4 for males and 35.7 for females that Himmelfarb and Murrel found in their 1984 study of the elderly residents of that Kentucky community. Moreover, while only 20% of elderly in that sample had anxiety scores that exceeded the psychiatric cutoff, 32.8% of the elderly in the Israeli sample did.

Thus, whether one looks at the figures in terms of psychiatric cutoff points or of means, Israel's elderly citizens, those who had not gone through the Holocaust as well as those who did, show markedly greater trait anxiety than the elderly residents of Himmelfarb and Murrel's Kentucky community. As we noted above, Israel's elderly have seen more than their share of upheavals, and the relatively high trait anxiety of the nonsurvivors may be an outcome of that.

The high trait anxiety of Israel's elderly in comparison with that of their Kentucky age mates highlights the impact of the Holocaust on the survivors. The survivors' response to the Gulf War was measured not against that of people who have led largely uneventful lives but against that of people who have had difficult life experiences and relatively high trait anxiety of their own. The fact that the trait anxiety of the Holocaust survivors was even higher is yet another indication of the pervasive, lasting impact of that cataclysm.

The survivors of the Holocaust were subjected not only to the threat of death, but to a massive onslaught against their integrity as human beings. Candidates for genocide, they were subjected to years of concerted German efforts to dehumanize them. In that context, they suffered starvation, forced transports, delocalization, labor, systematic humiliation and degradation, separation from their loved ones, uprooting, and the decimation of their families through violent, unnatural deaths. The experiences of those who survived the concentration camps and those who survived in hiding, in the partisans, or through flight to places beyond the Nazi reach are somewhat different from one another, and our sample was too small to find any potential differentiation in the impact of these modes of survival. But all the survivors share losses of enormous magnitude and, in contrast to Ra'anan Weitz and others in Israel who could bear arms in their own defense, are burdened by a legacy of profound helplessness in the face of an overwhelming, malevolent power.

# 7

# The Evacuees

Most of this book focuses on groups of Israelis who may have been frightened during the Gulf War, but sustained no losses or injuries. This chapter looks at the war's only direct casualties: the people who were evacuated from their homes following Scud strikes. These people suffered various degrees of injury to their persons and property. Some came out with bruises and scratches and with minor damage to their homes—broken windows and doors that could be easily replaced, cracked walls that needed little more than plaster and paint to put them right. Others, fewer, were trapped under the rubble of fallen ceilings and/or lost their homes and most of their worldly goods. One person was killed, leaving his son and 51-year-old wife to start life anew without him, without their home, and with barely a memento of their life as a whole family (Kedem, 1991a).

Against the backdrop of this century's many human-made horrors and of the continuing brutalities of the numerous ideological and ethnic wars that are raging as this book is being written, even this damage, the worst that the Gulf War inflicted, was relatively minor. About 9,000 homes in the Tel Aviv and Ramat Gan area were damaged by Scuds or flying debris, and 1,500 people temporarily evacuated to hotels at government expense. But within a few weeks, by the beginning of March 1993, a third of the damaged structures had been repaired, and two-thirds of the evacuees, as they were called, were out of the hotels and back under their own roofs, with relatives, or in rented apartments, also at government expenses. All in all, only 120 buildings were condemned to demolition, most of them old two-story houses in slum neighborhoods (Grinblatt, 1991).

But if from the lofty perspective of numbers the damage was contained and most of it soon repaired, from the perspective of the individuals who found themselves out on the street one winter night, before the buses came to take them to the hotels where they were put up, the picture was very different. The home, according to Ben Yakar (1991), is not only a physical structure. It is also a symbol: a symbol of safety, of security, of the inviolability of the self. For every person whose home was seriously damaged or destroyed, the loss had a deep and personal meaning in addition to its substantial material significance. Ben Yakar tells of a young married couple for whom the destruction of their apartment signified the futility of their relationship; of a man for whom the strike was reminiscent of his flight as a child from a bombing raid in World War II; of an elderly Holocaust survivor who salvaged from the rubble of her scudded apartment an old silver spoon and an invitation to a social event that linked her to her past and place in society; and of others. A newspaper article written at the time tells of a woman whose son had died the year before and whose mementos of him were all buried under the debris of her house (Kedem, 1991b). The missiles thus struck at different points in the victims' lives, and to each the damage had its own particular meaning. In this, the victims of the Scud attacks are much like the victims of other mass disasters, who not only must rebuild the physical structures of their lives but also must deal with the many psychological reverberations and implications of their experience.

The actual missile attack and the destruction of their homes was only part of the experience of the evacuees, as they were called. It was followed by their evacuation by bus to hotels, where they received temporary shelter, and by the process of physical reconstruction.

Both the Tel Aviv and Ramat Gan municipalities were very efficient in organizing emergency accommodations for all those whose homes were damaged in the missile strikes. In both cities, buses were promptly dispatched to the missile sites, and all those who could not or would not return to their homes were offered temporary hotel accommodations. This gave the victims a certain respite from the need to find shelter while they regained their bearings and set about seeing to the repair of the damage, where possible. According to reports, the evacuees generally arrived at the hotels in a state of shock. Some received tranquilizers from doctors who made themselves available. Many expressed a variety of Scud-induced fears, including fear of being alone, fear that they were being pursued by missiles, and fear of another strike. Buses were also provided at the hotels to take the residents back to their neighborhoods to assess the damage and see what could be salvaged. The children were picked up and driven to school. Representatives of various government offices, including the National Insurance Institute and welfare and property tax bureaus, came with forms for the residents to fill out (Nevo,

1991). These services enabled the evacuees to go back to work or to supervise the repair of their homes. For those who did neither, however, a kind of malaise set in. "Life became breakfast, lunch and dinner, in between aimless wandering around the hotel or just sitting in the lobby smoking cigarettes. For some, the lack of intimacy and the unfamiliar food posed a problem. In some of the hotels the guests' restlessness began to show: lobby furniture was vandalized, lamps disappeared, cigarette burns in the upholstery" (Felldman, 1991).

The physical rebuilding started fairly soon after the attacks. In the immediate aftermath of each strike, those who could not or would not stay in their homes were transported by bus to one of several hotels, where they were temporarily housed. Within a few days, one or more family members were back at the site of their home to ascertain the damage and to salvage what could be saved, and then to start on the reconstruction. In this, the victims of the strikes received government assistance, including reimbursement for inexpensive repairs (up to NIS 2000, about $600), larger repairs made by government contractors, and compensation for their losses by the National Insurance Institute. The motive behind the assistance was the same as that behind compensation to wounded soldiers and to the families of fallen soldiers: that the society as a whole must share the costs of war damage.

The sting in the ointment was that the implementation of the assistance inevitably brought the victims—who were anxious, on edge, and sometimes still dazed and numb—into confrontation with the intricate bureaucracy that was mobilized to help them. They had to fill out endless forms, wait in long lines in crowded government offices, come back the next day with more information, and so forth. For the Property Tax Office, they had to declare on paper the damage to their home, its contents, and their car, which then sent its own people out to check and verify before contractors were dispatched to make repairs and compensation paid for lost belongings. Given the mass of claims, this inevitably took time, and all the more so because claims totaling millions of dollars could not reasonably be accepted at face value. The delay, the questioning, and the inevitable disagreements about the real value of the lost objects made fertile ground for frustration and friction. So did the fact that the compensation was partial (jewelry, art works, and so on were excluded) and not always commensurate with the real current costs of replacing the objects. In addition some of the victims felt that they had been pressured into making hasty, incomplete declarations while they were still in a state of shock, and were not being fairly compensated as a result, or that inexperienced appraisers who had been hired for the emergency undervalued their losses.

The nature and scope of the repairs to be made on each apartment was decided by a committee, and the timetable was set by the various contractors the municipalities hired to do the work. The contractors, who typically worked on several projects simultaneously, did not necessarily adhere to the schedule, and the construction workers did not always arrive at the hour or even on the day they said they would. Evacuees who came from the hotels to oversee the repairs could be left waiting for days in their damaged apartments before the workers, among them Russian immigrants who had never worked in construction before, arrived (Chen, Y., 1991).

Thus, the entire experience of the evacuees, not only the missile attack but also the work of reconstruction, could leave them feeling helpless and not in control of their lives.

## OMISSIONS IN STUDIES TO DATE

The delayed and long-term effects of psychic trauma have been documented in a large variety of settings. Most of the studies, however, were conducted many months or years after the traumatic event (for example, Kluznik, Speed, van Valkenburg, & Margraw, 1986; Kulka, et al., 1988). In contrast, there are relatively few studies to date of *early* responses to traumatic stress and relatively few studies following up the victims of such stress over time. There are not even any standard criteria for the assessment of acute stress reactions.

These are unfortunate omissions. The few studies there are on the subject suggest that acute stress reactions both are extremely labile (Solomon, Mikulincer, & Benbenishty, 1989a; Yizhaki, Solomon, & Kotler, 1991) and have a different clinical picture from later reactions and should thus be considered a distinct clinical entity (Middleton & Raphael, 1990; Rahe, 1988). Moreover, there is some evidence that the initial response to stress may be highly predictive of future adjustment. Prior studies by my colleagues and myself (Solomon 1989a) of Israeli combat soldiers in the 1982 Lebanon War showed that those who sustained acute combat stress reactions (CSR) on the front were four to five times more likely than comparable non-CSR soldiers to develop chronic posttraumatic stress disorder (PTSD) in the three years following the war. Studies with combat veterans also suggest that some early symptoms may be more predictive than others of future problems (Laufer, Frey-Wouters, & Gallops, 1985; Mikulincer, Solomon & Benbenbishty, 1988), and that the more symptoms there are early on the more likely are problems in the future (Solomon, Benbenishty, & Mikulincer, 1988). A better understanding of the immediate responses to war stress should thus facilitate identifying persons at high risk for long-term PTSD.

## REACTIONS TO THE SCUDS: EXPOSURE AND SOCIOECONOMIC CLASS

Had I been left to my own devices, I am not at all sure that I would have made a study of the victims of the Scud strikes. Whatever the scientific merits of the subject, the act of distributing questionnaires to people who just lost their homes would have seemed more than a bit callous. The study came about as a result of two telephone calls that made it possible for me to combine the pursuit of scientific interest with helping out some of the evacuees. The first was from Professor Nathanial Laor, director of the Psychiatric Clinic at Ramat Gan. He had been asked by the Tel Aviv municipality to examine the evacuees at the various hotels to see whether any of them needed mental health assistance. Since the staff at the clinic were not geared to working in mass crises and, moreover, many of its personnel were either at home minding their kids or out of town altogether, he asked me to help out. The second call came a few days later, with a similar request from Ora Hadar and David Weiler, who headed a team of social workers who had volunteered to assist in the Acadia Hotel in Herzelia. The data were collected as part of a needs assessment at the two sites, where the psychologists and social workers administered the questionnaires in the course of interviewing the evacuees.

The study presented below (Solomon, et al., 1993) was carried out in two stages, the first a week after the evacuation of the subjects to two sites following serious damage to their apartments during missile strikes, the second a year later.

### The Immediate Response

The first phase of the study aimed at ascertaining the nature of acute symptomatology and examining the impact of background variable, level of exposure, and postdisaster environment on the immediate stress response. Two groups were studied: 69 evacuees from a lower-class Tel Aviv neighborhood and 51 evacuees from a middle-class neighborhood in the adjacent city of Ramat Gan. A battery of self-report questionnaires was administered individually to each of the subjects in their hotels a week after their evacuation. The questionnaires tapped the evacuees' socioeconomic status and postrecovery environment, on the one hand, and their acute stress responses after the missile attacks, on the other.

### Background Variables

The two groups had the same ratio of males to females (38% and 62%, respectively). But the Tel Aviv group was somewhat younger than the Ramat Gan group, had more children per family, and reported poorer living conditions prior to evacuation.

### Level of Exposure

The two groups reported similar levels of exposure to the stressor: 83% stated that they had experienced a high or very high level of threat during the missile attack; 64% believed that they had been in danger of death or injury; 27% reported that their homes were totally destroyed; and 25% had been in close proximity to casualties.

### Postdisaster Environment

This factor has not been included in any of the other studies of the Gulf War that I know of. Though there are indications in the literature that the postdisaster environment may be critical to whether initial stress reactions pass or, alternatively, crystallize into chronic PTSD (Hoiberg & McCaughey, 1984), it was not generally relevant to the particular concerns of those studies and, in any case, would have been extremely difficult if not impossible to define operationally. With regard to the evacuees, it so happened that the approaches of the Tel Aviv and Ramat Gan municipalities who took care of them after the missile strikes were poles apart, so that each could be clearly distinguished and its impact assessed.

Most of the Ramat Gan evacuees were put up in a four-star hotel similar to the one described below and received considerable attention from a host of municipal workers and volunteers, as well as from the mayor of the city. The Tel Aviv evacuees were put up in a "flea hole" where they were regarded with mistrust and suspicion, as though they were out to exploit their misery for secondary gains. The difference is aptly described in a newspaper article:

> A Na'amat [a women's organization] volunteer who spent two days working with the evacuees in a Tel Aviv hotel reports that there is a very unpleasant atmosphere and no personal attention. The evacuees are very aggressive and so is the mayor. At the

Kfar Hamaccabia Hotel, the [Ramat Gan] evacuees have a special storeroom of used
and new clothes, a synagogue, kindergarten, nurse, doctor, and mental health unit.
A delux evacuation. On every floor there are two sealed rooms equipped with a TV,
mineral water, air conditioner and radio. After every alarm the psychologists come
round to calm down the evacuees. They were given wash kits and slippers, and get
three meals a day and free tea and coffee and cake on the patio in the afternoon.
Their rooms are cleaned and sheets are changed every day, and the laundry is done.
They will eventually have to pay for the phone calls.

At the Tal hotel in Tel Aviv, the evacuees got box lunches. . . . The food was so
bad that a catering service was brought in, but at three shekels a head per meal,
which for some families was financially impossible. The evacuees send their laundry
to a laundromat or wash it by themselves and hang the clothes in the hallway. . . .
Phone calls only from a public phone. . . . Sheets and towels are changed every so
often. . . . Every room is sealed so people smoke in the halls. Free coffee and tea
were put out only the first few days; then the hotel management told them to bring
a thermos from home. What home? (Shabi, 1991)

The Ramat Gan evacuees in this study were at the Acadia Hotel in
Herzelia, but the conditions and atmosphere there were much the same
as those at the Kfar Maccabia described in this article. Having visited
various hotels where the evacuees stayed, I can vouch for the general
tenor of this description. The feeling among the Tel Aviv evacuees who
were put up in low-grade hotels was that if they had been from a wealth-
ier part of the city they would have received better treatment (Trabelski
& Rosolio, 1991).

The difference was reflected in the two groups' evaluations of their
postdisaster environment. Significantly more of the Ramat Gan than the
Tel Aviv subjects viewed the evacuation efforts as efficient (74% versus
66%), and more than twice as many of them rated their hotel accommodations as very good (59% versus 21%).

The evacuees' reactions to the missile strikes were assessed by a number of different measures. This was done in order to distinguish between
what is known to be specifically trauma-induced symptomatology and
general symptomatology. The *Impact of Event Scale* (IES; Horowitz, Wilner, & Alvarez, 1979) was used to assess the standard intrusion and avoidance tendencies following exposure to traumatic events. The *Symptom
Checklist 90 Revised* (SCL-90-R; Derogatis, 1977) was used to obtain both
global measures of general psychiatric symptomatology and specific
symptom pictures. In addition, subjects from Tel Aviv completed the
*State-Trait Anxiety Inventory* (Spielberger et al., 1970), and subjects from
Ramat Gan completed a *PTSD Inventory* based on DSM-III-R criteria.

The basic finding was that a week after the missile strikes, most
evacuees showed a very high level of distress in all the measures. Both
the state and trait anxiety scores of the Ramat Gan evacuees exceeded

those reported by Saigh (1988) among Lebanese university students one week after heavy shelling of Beirut. The SCL-90-R scores showing general emotional distress were also extremely high. The scores on each of the three global indices—the Global Severity index (GSI), which is the average intensity of all 90 symptoms; the Positive Symptom Total (PST), which is the number of positively endorsed symptoms; and the Positive Symptom Distress Index (PSDI), which is the average intensity of the endorsed symptoms—all hovered around the norm for psychiatric outpatients (Derogatis, 1977). And on four of the separate symptoms scales (somatization, anxiety, hostility, and phobic anxiety), the evacuees from the lower socioeconomic class scored higher.

What is most striking, however, is the very high level of PTSD symptomatology found. A full 80% of those assessed on the PTSD Inventory displayed a constellation of symptoms consistent with DSM-III-R criteria for the disorder. While a formal diagnosis of PTSD cannot be considered so soon after a traumatic event (according to the DSM-III-R, a minimum six-month duration for symptoms is required), the finding does indicate that the vast majority of people respond to traumatic events with a level of stress and a constellation of symptoms that would be deemed pathological if they persisted. It suggests that even if the symptoms may abate with time, and even though not everyone who manifests them during or soon after a disaster develops full-blown PTSD, the PTSD constellation is an almost universal and entirely normal immediate response to extreme stress.

This suggestion is reinforced by the findings on the IES, which both groups of evacuees filled out. As noted above, the IES is a specific measure of trauma. It taps the frequency of the intrusion of trauma-related memories, images, dreams, and so forth into consciousness and the person's attempts to avoid such recollections by such maneuvers as putting them out of mind and avoiding people, places, and activities that recall the traumatic event. The measure is thus indicative of people's continuing absorption with the traumatic event, whether through its unwanted intrusion into their psyches or through their efforts to escape, block, or repel those intrusions.

Both groups seem to have scored high on this measure. In contrast to DSM-III-R PTSD criteria, the IES has no cutoff score distinguishing high from low levels. However, both groups of Scud evacuees endorsed almost as many intrusion (Tel Aviv: 3.02; Ramat Gan: 2.63) and avoidance (Tel Aviv: 1.71; Ramat Gan: 1.92) responses as reported by Israeli combat soldiers diagnosed with PTSD one and three years after the Lebanon War (Solomon, 1993).

Moreover, there were no significant differences in the scores of the two groups on the IES, while there were on the SCL-90-R measure of general symptomatology. In all three of its global indices, the GSI, the PSD, and the PSDI, the lower socioeconomic Tel Aviv group revealed significantly more extensive and more severe psychopathology than the middle-class Ramat Gan group. As can be seen in Figure 7.1, they also scored higher on each of the measure's nine symptom categories. Set against these differences in general psychiatric symptomatology, the similarity in specifically trauma-related symptomatology further indicates that the trauma-related symptoms, in fact, do have their roots in the traumatic event and not in the victim's background or personality, as has sometimes been claimed (Blank, 1985).

Indeed, further analyses confirmed that the trauma-related symptomatology and the general symptomatology stemmed from different sources. Findings showed that the general psychiatric symptomatology (as measured by the SCL-90-R) was explained primarily by the background variables, especially the adequacy of the respondent's housing,

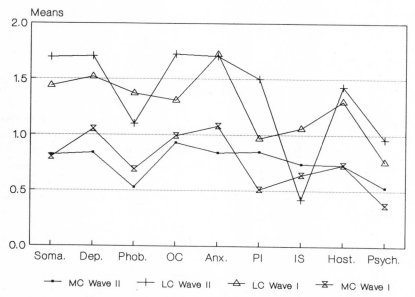

**Figure 7.1.** Means of SCL-90-R subscales by study group and time of assessment. *Key:* MC Wave I—middle-class evacuees, during the war; LC Wave I—lower-class evacuees, during the war; MC Wave II—middle-class evacuees, 2nd year; LC Wave II—lower-class evacuees, 2nd year; Soma.—somatization; Dep.—depression; Phob.—phobic anxiety; OC—obsessive–compulsive; Anx.—anxiety; PI—paranoid ideation; IS—interpersonal sensitivity; Host.—hostility; Psych.—psychotism.

which accounted for 17% of the variance. Level of exposure, as measured by perception of threat, perception of danger of death or injury, degree of damage to the respondent's home, and proximity to casualties, explained less of the variance, 8.9%, while postdisaster variables contributed only 0.9%. In contrast, a total of 34.2% of the variance on the intrusion scale of the IES was explained by the conjunction of the level of exposure (27.5%) and the postdisaster variables (6.7%), and none by the background variables.

The findings of high distress in the aftermath of the disaster are consistent with eyewitness reports of the evacuees in their hotels. According to Etti Friedman, a municipal social worker who worked with a group of Ramat Gan evacuees at the Acadia Hotel in Hertzelia, the evacuees were initially "in a state of shock." The day they arrived, they were disoriented, insisting that everything was all right and that there were no problems. But within 24 hours signs of anxiety surfaced. Entire families hung out in the lobby or walked about the hallways rather than be alone in their rooms. Children who had assumed parental roles and mothers who had tried to be strong for their families broke down. Some evacuees were afraid to go out at night and afraid to part even temporarily from other family members (Miron, 1991).

**One Year Later**

One year later, a follow-up assessment was made to ascertain the long-term effects of the missile strikes. This time, six groups of subjects were examined: two groups of evacuees from the same two neighborhoods as the subjects in the first phase of the study; two groups of nonevacuees from those same neighborhoods (that is, people who were directly exposed to the missile strikes but whose homes were not directly hit and thus were not evacuated to hotels; and two groups of controls, one from a lower-class neighborhood, the other from a middle-class neighborhood in Jerusalem, a city where no missiles struck and which was not even on the missile trajectory. Both evacuee groups included a sizable number of subjects who had participated in the study the year before.

The groups represented three different levels of exposure and two different socioeconomic classes. The purpose of this division was to gauge the impact of exposure, on the one hand, and of socioeconomic background, on the other, to responses to traumatic events. The evacuees were defined as high exposure, the nonevacuees from the scudded neighborhoods as medium exposure, and the Jerusalemites as low exposure. Data collected on the respondents' wartime experiences coincided with these definitions. The evacuees from the scudded neighborhoods, whether middle or lower class, rated the danger they were in as highest, reported the most serious damage to their homes, and endorsed the greatest proximity to casualties. The Jerusalemites made the lowest endorsements of these items, and the nonevacuees in the scudded neighborhoods reported levels in between, though at least a third of them left their homes for relatives' homes or hotels.

The participants filled out the same questionnaires as in the first phase: the PTSD Inventory and the IES, which tapped specifically trauma-related symptomatology; the SCL-90-R; and Spielberger's State-Trait Anxiety Inventory. They also filled out questionnaires gauging the extent of their exposure to the missile strikes, their current family closeness, their postdisaster functioning, and their feeling of need for medical and psychological help.

Comparisons over time show that although trauma-related symptomatology declined somewhat, it was still quite high in both groups. PTSD rates in the middle-class evacuees fell from 80% to under 60%. While numerically significant, this reduction still left over half the evacuees with PTSD a year after their homes were bombed. Similarly, the mean number of IES intrusion responses also declined only modestly. Though both the middle- and lower-class evacuees endorsed fewer intrusion symptoms (2.28 and 2.62, respectively) than they had the previous year, the mean intrusion score of the lower socioeconomic strata evacuees still resembled that of PTSD combat soldiers three years after the Lebanon War (Solomon, 1993). Moreover, in both groups, and most prominently in the middle-class evacuees, the decline in intrusion was matched by an increase of avoidance. In short, a considerable proportion of the evacuees continued to suffer from trauma-related symptomatology a year after the missile strikes that damaged or destroyed their homes.

They also continued to suffer from general psychiatric symptomatology as measured by the SCL-90-R. As can be seen from Figure 7.1, there was at best a very minor decline in general symptomatology in either of the groups. What is salient is that the substantial difference in the level of symptomatology of the middle and lower socioeconomic strata that was noted immediately after their evacuation was extant a year later as well. Once again, the evacuees from the poorer neighborhood endorsed a substantially higher level of symptoms in every category than their middle-class counterparts with roughly similar exposure to the missile attacks.

Comparison of all six groups at the one-year mark reveals a rough dose-response pattern combined or tempered with the strong impact of socioeconomic status.

*PTSD status* a year after the war was directly related first to level of exposure and second to socioeconomic class. As can be seen from Figure 7.2, the evacuees had the highest PTSD rates, the nonevacuees in the scudded area the next to highest, and the Jerusalemites, who were in little danger of attack, the lowest. Then within each level of exposure, the respondents from the lower-class neighborhoods generally had higher rates of PTSD than those from the middle-class neighborhoods. The difference was greatest among the evacuees, somewhat less but still substantial among the evacuees, somewhat less but still substantial among the scudded nonevacuees, and practically nonperceptible among the Jerusalemites.

The pattern was much the same for the three *symptom categories in the PTSD syndrome*—intrusion, avoidance, and arousal. Endorsement of

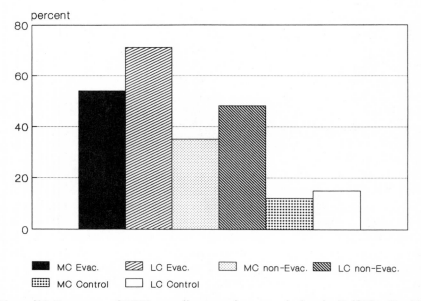

**Figure 7.2.** Percentage of PTSD according to study groups during the Gulf War. *Key:* MC Evac.—middle-class evacuees; LC Evac.—lower-class evacuees; MC non-Evac.—middle-class nonevacuees; LC non-Evac.—lower-class nonevacuees; MC Control—middle-class controls; LC Control—lower-class controls.

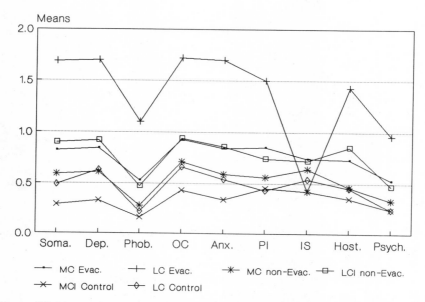

**Figure 7.3.** Means of SCL-90-R subscales by study group during the Gulf War. *Key:* MC Evac.—middle-class evacuees; LC Evac.—lower-class evacuees; MC non-Evac.—middle-class nonevacuees; LC non-Evac.—lower-class nonevacuees; MC Control—middle-class controls; LC Control—lower-class controls; Soma.—somatization; Dep.—depression; Phob.—phobic anxiety; OC—obsessive–compulsive; Anx.—anxiety; PI—paranoid ideation; IS—interpersonal sensitivity; Host.—hostility; Psych.—psychotism.

each of these symptom categories reflected the level of exposure. However, here the impact of socioeconomic status was pronounced only among the evacuees but not among the scudded nonevacuees or the Jerusalemites.

With minor variations, the pattern was also similar on all the other measures.

On the *IES*, the highest endorsements on both intrusion and avoidance were made by the evacuees, the middle by the nonevacuees form the scudded areas, and the lowest by the Jerusalemites. Socioeconomic status played a role only among the evacuees; those from the lower-class neighborhood scored highest on both intrusion and avoidance. There were no class differences in the reports of the scudded nonevacuees or of the Jerusalemites.

On the *SCL-90-R*, the lower-class evacuees recorded the greatest general distress. They had the highest Global Severity score and en-

dorsed the most symptoms. As can be seen on Figure 7.3, the lower
socioeconomic strata evacuees reported substantially higher levels on
each of the nine symptom categories than any of the other groups.
Moreover, within each exposure group, the lower-class subjects endorsed
higher symptom levels than their middle-class counterparts.

Figure 7.3 also reveals that the symptoms of the middle-class group
in each of the exposure categories corresponded quite closely to the
symptom levels among the lower-class subjects in the exposure category
just below. There is virtually no difference between the symptom endorsement of the middle-class evacuees and the lower-class nonevacuees
from Tel Aviv, and similarly little difference between the endorsements
of the middle-class nonevacuees and the lower-class Jerusalemites. The
difference between the lower- and middle-class subjects in each category
exceeds these. This pattern provides a clear illustration of the protection
from stress that their middle-class status provided. Indeed, of all the
groups, the middle-class Jerusalemites tended to make the lowest endorsements of most of the symptoms.

On the *State-Trait Anxiety Inventory*, the lower-class evacuees had both
the highest state anxiety and the highest trait anxiety, indicating their
response both to the trauma of their evacuation and to the conditions of
their lives. When it came to the middle-class evacuees, however, only
their state anxiety was substantially higher than in the control groups.
Their trait anxiety was similar to that of the nonevacuees and higher
only than that of the middle-class Jerusalemites.

On the measure of *Family Closeness*, which was devised for this study
to determine feelings of closeness, mutual help, family members' enjoyment of each others' company, shared decision making, and so forth,
lower-class evacuees had lower scores than middle-class evacuees, indicating either that their evacuation undermined their family closeness
more or, more likely, that these families were less close to begin with. In
either case, the finding suggests that they were less likely than their
middle-class counterparts to benefit from family support in the postat-
tack adjustment period.

Endorsements of *need for medical and mental health assistance* also reflected the impact of both exposure and socioeconomic status. In general, endorsement of the need for medical help was highest among the
evacuees, somewhat less among the nonevacuees from the same neighborhoods, and significantly less among the Jerusalemites. In the high-
exposure area, a full 57% of the lower-class evacuees stated that they felt
the need for medical help as opposed to 31% of the middle-class evacuees, though there was no such gap in the endorsements of the non-

evacuees (25% of both groups or of the Jerusalemites 6% and 3%, for middle- and lower-class subjects, respectively).

The pattern was even more pronounced in the need for mental health assistance. This need was positively endorsed by 50% of the lower-class evacuees in contrast to only 17% of the middle-class evacuees. Among the nonevacuees, the rates plummeted to around 10% in both groups, and fell still further among the Jerusalemites of both socio-economic levels.

Finally, much the same pattern emerged in *changes in functioning* since the Gulf War. On the whole, the evacuees, and especially those from the lower-class neighborhood, reported the highest rate of negative changes in overall functioning (family, work, leisure time), the greatest impairment of ability to work, the greatest increase in physical difficulties at work, the most work days lost as a result of the war, the greatest decline in the importance they attached to their work, the greatest overall sense of impaired goals at work, the greatest increase in social problems at work, and the greatest increase in cigarette consumption. On all of these items, the pattern of descent was much the same as that in the various other measures of psychological well-being. Only alcohol consumption was apparently unaffected by the war, which is consistent with previous findings on trauma survivors in Israel (for example, Solomon, 1993).

## SUMMARY AND CONCLUSIONS

Eight different measures tapping various aspects of the mental health of the victims of the Scud attacks during the Gulf War delineate a similar picture, with only minor variations.

To begin with, the findings show that the war left its mark on the Scud victims. A year later, it was still very much alive in the evacuees' high rates of PTSD and in their continuing struggle with intrusive wartime memories and their concomitant efforts to avoid them. In Chapter 2, we observed that the vast majority of the adult population coped well with the war. In chapter 5, we observed that very few children showed signs of distress a year after the war's end. Here we find that the victims of the Scud attacks were not so fortunate. Even though their level of distress was evidently lower than in the immediate aftermath of the war, the evacuees still showed both high trauma-related and high general psychiatric symptomatology.

Findings also show that the level of distress was related to the level of exposure. This was true both immediately after the missile strikes and a year later. On all the measures, the evacuees showed more trauma-related and general distress, higher state anxiety, greater feelings of need for medical and psychiatric assistance, and more negative changes in their family lives, leisure-time enjoyment, and work lives than the nonevacuees; the nonevacuees from the scudded neighborhoods showed somewhat less distress on these measures; and the non-scudded and nonendangered Jerusalemites showed the lowest levels of distress. In the descending pattern of distress, what we see is a clear and consistent dose response. This is consistent with findings of previous studies attesting to the impact of exposure on the distress ensuing from response to disasters and other traumatic experiences (for example, Pynoos, et al., 1987).

The findings also show a differential level of distress in the subjects from lower- and middle-class neighborhoods. In the immediate aftermath of the attacks, the distinction was revealed only in the trauma-related measures. A year later, it was also evident in the more general measures of psychological well-being. Apparently, personal differences are dwarfed around the time of a traumatic experience only to emerge later on.

In both the trauma-related and general psychiatric and functional measures, lower-class subjects fared worse than middle-class subjects. The distinction was most substantial among the evacuees, where it ran through all the assessments. In measure after measure, the lower-class evacuees showed considerably more distress than their middle-class counterparts, even though the two groups were exposed to a similar level of external stress. Indeed, the lower-class evacuees consistently stood out as the group that suffered most from the Scud attacks.

Their greater suffering in the wake of their evacuations can be attributed to either or both of two factors that have been amply noted in the literature. One is prior vulnerability linked to their socioeconomic class. There is repeated evidence in the literature that people of low socioeconomic status suffer from higher rates of psychiatric disorders than those of higher status (for example, Dohrenwend & Dohrenwend, 1969; Dohrenwend, et al., 1992). One of the various explanations offered is the "social drift hypothesis," which holds that it is largely the people who are poorly equipped to cope with life to begin with who are found in the lower socioeconomic ranks of society (Dohrenwend & Dohrenwend, 1969; Dohrenwend et al., 1992). A contrasting account is offered by the "social causation hypothesis," which maintains that the intense strains of life at the bottom of the socioeconomic ladder exhaust people's coping resources and thus render them more vulnerable to pathology, especially in the face of adversity (Dohrenwend & Dohrenwend, 1969; Dohrenwend et al., 1992).

The other possible factor is the differential recovery environment. As described above, the middle-class evacuees were transported to four-star hotels where they were treated with a great deal of care and consideration, while the lower-class evacuees were brought to "flea holes" where they were begrudged and treated with suspicion. Moreover, it can be assumed that once their homes were repaired, the middle-class evacuees returned to more spacious and pleasing abodes than their lower-class counterparts. The finding that portions of the variance in symptoms shortly after the attacks derived from the nature of the subjects' housing and postdisaster environment highlights the importance of a supportive recovery environment for the mental health of disaster victims.

The mental health distinction between the lower- and middle-class subjects consistently decreases with declining level of exposure. In some measures, the distinction was evident only among the evacuees. In a few measures it appeared also among the evacuees from the scudded neighborhoods, but was much narrower. In none of the measures was it evident among the nonscudded Jerusalemites. This pattern suggest that poor socioeconomic status is associated with damage to mental health mainly when extremely intense external pressures add to the pressures inherent in poverty, or when poverty adds its pressures to those of extreme stressors.

The findings of low distress among the Jerusalemites is consistent with the findings in Chapter 2 of Israelis' generally adaptive coping with the pressures of the war and its overhanging threat. Those findings suggest that the war had little if any long-term adverse psychological effect on people whose homes and neighborhoods were not hit by Scuds. The 10% rate of PTSD found among the Jerusalemites corresponds to PTSD rates both in the general population of Israel (Dohrenwend et al., 1992) and among untreated Israeli combat veterans (Solomon, 1993). This correspondence is further evidence that whatever psychological effect the war may have had on the general population in the short term soon passed.

# 8

# Psychiatric Patients
## Stressed, Buffered, or Forced to Cope?

It is commonly assumed that people respond to disasters and other intense stressors in keeping with their emotional health prior to their exposure. As Gibbs (1989) puts it in her review of factors that mediate between disaster and psychopathology, "One would expect that more disturbed individuals would have poorer coping skills, and thus would be less able to cope with the severe stress involved" (p. 499). In this popular view, psychiatric patients and even people in psychotherapy or counseling would constitute a high-risk population.

But is the assumption supported by facts? The difficulty of obtaining prior data on any group of individuals and the various difficulties of doing research on the mentally ill both make the question problematic to answer. It is not surprising that there has been little empirical study of the reactions of the mentally ill to disaster and even fewer studies of their reactions in wartime. We have almost no information that would enable prediction of either their needs or responses in situations of collective life threat, such as the Gulf War was. At most, the literature suggests three possible scenarios: that such life threat would exacerbate their illness, have no effect on their condition, or improve their condition.

The most pessimistic scenario is based on the life-change model (Dohrenwend & Dohrenwend, 1974), which regards any change as stressful and potentially harmful. The model holds that extreme stress triggers or aggravates illness or unmasks latent disease processes, mental no less than physical. The scenario based on this model would predict that the mentally ill would respond to war with regression and exacerbation of symptoms. Schulberg (1974) suggests that adaptation to disaster will vary with the person's vulnerability to the event, and that while the normal adult is highly adaptive, the chronic schizophrenic exhibits minimal tolerance for many types of stress.

The second scenario is based on the view that mental illness serves as a buffer against external stress so would *not be affected* by it. According to Freud, the libidinal energy of the schizophrenic is removed from his social surroundings and invested in his internal world, to be projected onto the environment in the form of delusions and bizarre thoughts (Bendor, Gelkopf, & Sigal, 1993). Rofe (1989) hypothesizes that while mental illness may develop as a means of coping with internal personal stressors, it does not develop in response to universal external stressors. Rofe cites evidence to the effect that although some concentration camp survivors, patients with incurable diseases, and prisoners in Soviet labor camps, all of whom were exposed to extreme external stress, suffer from anxiety-related or neurotic symptoms, they do not generally develop psychoses. The findings suggest that while intense external stress may lead to emotional disorders, those are specific in kind and limited in intensity. It does not produce psychosis. More direct support for the view that the mentally ill would not be affected by extreme stress is provided by Bromet, Schulberg, and Dunn's (1982) comparison of the mental health status of psychiatric patients in the vicinity of the Three Mile Island nuclear plant following the accident with that of patients living in an area where a similar plant was located. This study found no difference in the anxiety or depressive episodes in the two groups and no difference in the severity of their symptoms following the disaster.

The third scenario is based on the view that intense external stress may distract the mentally ill from their inner turmoil and force them to attend to the demands of reality. The scenario here would be that the Gulf War would actually *improve* the functioning of the mentally ill.

This scenario is consistent with Weil's (1975) observations of Israeli psychiatric patients in Rambam Hospital in Haifa during the 1973 Yom Kippur War. To make room for possible military casualties, 30 psychiatric patients had to be sent home at the start of the war, even though in the opinion of the staff they still required hospitalization. This created natural conditions in which their wartime functioning could be systematically studied. When they were reexamined 10 months after the war, it was found that of the 30 patients formally in the hospital, only 4 (2 of whom had a prior history of multiple hospitalizations) had to be hospitalized. All the others managed on their own. Moreover, Weil also reports that there was a drastic reduction in psychiatric admissions during the eight weeks of the war, down to 51 from 110 in the same period the year before. Weil explains these findings with the suggestion that during national crises in Israel, even the mentally ill are able to put aside their personal problems. They leave the hospital as their contribution to the war effort, and at home they try their best not to impose additional burdens. Their families, meanwhile, are more ready to be kind and accepting. The scenario is also consistent with the well-documented decline in psychiatric admissions during wartime (Weil, 1975). Both sets of findings suggest that in face of strong external stress, the mentally ill manage to organize themselves and to adapt to the demands of the environment.

Which of these scenarios applied during the Gulf War? What was the impact of the collective threat on the mentally ill?

The issue received considerable attention during the war both in the media and in several major psychiatric institutions in Israel, where members of the professional staff launched their own investigations. To answer our question, we looked at the various reports, both newspaper articles and professional papers. The reports vary in size and scope. Some are clinical observations of a few individuals; others are more systematic studies of larger samples. In this chapter we begin by looking at the clinical impressions, then examine the research findings.

## CLINICAL FINDINGS

### Therapists' Impressions

In terms of what actually happened in Israel, the Gulf War can be considered largely a war of nerves. The vast majority of people incurred no actual physical damage. But the constant threat, the repeated alarms, the multitudinous disruptions of daily life, the hanging suspense, the suspension or subordination of other concerns, and the concerted focus of people's thoughts on the war gave it a substantial psychological dimension. As long as there was food in the stores and power in the lines, and as long as injuries were limited and war deaths were few, the war remained essentially a psychological event. This fact was sensed and conveyed by the media. For along with the flood of news broadcasts, bulletins, and analyses, a great deal of media attention was devoted to psychological issues: how the threat was affecting people emotionally, how to keep calm, how to cope with frightened children, and so forth. It was also incorporated and expressed in actions and policies, such as the numerous telephone hotlines set up by various organizations (the army, the Tel Aviv Municipality, and psychological clinics) to give emergency emotional support to troubled callers.

In short, the Gulf War projected psychological issues into consciousness. Responsive to the interest, the jornalist Aviva Kroll (1991) interviewed several therapists to get their impressions of the effect of the war on their patients. The article she wrote describes a range of responses.

A large number of long-term psychotherapy patients apparently put their problems on hold and stopped going to their regular therapy sessions. The temporary cessation of therapy was not dissimilar to the suspension of other activities during the war, and seems to have been motivated at least in part by a disinclination to venture out any more than necessary. Other reasons mentioned include the dwarfing of personal problems by the larger problems of the war, the difficulty of grappling with painful psychological issues in addition to the pressing issues of existence precipitated by the war, and the high cost of therapy when some people's incomes were dwindling.

If those patients were able to cope with their personal difficulties on their own for the duration of the war, certain types of patients, the article suggests, actually benefited from the crisis. People with paranoid inclinations are the most often mentioned. Others include patients with constricted functioning or dependent needs. The psychologist Noga Dim, of the Machon Ya'ad, a psychotherapy and counseling clinic in Tel Aviv, expresses the opinion that the more troubled of her patients were the ones who benefited most, and describes how:

> I discovered that some patients, especially the more troubled ones, pull themselves together and feel better: people with paranoid anxiety, for example. Everyone's reality is more paranoid today. Who would have believed a year ago that we'd have missles flying over our heads? The paranoids' fantasy of threat and persecution materialized. So now they can feel connected to reality and need not feel the conflict they felt when they were considered strange or different. Now they feel part of things: it's normal now to be paranoid, to feel persecuted, and to behave defensively.
>
> Also, people whose functioning is generally constricted and defensive, who only go out to work and come straight home again, feel better now. Their low activity level is in keeping with the restricted activity level that is the norm now. No one expects people to go out or be creative now. We're expected to be more concrete and practical—gas mask and sealed room. It's a less complex lifestyle, which creates less stress for these people.
>
> For dependent people, too, the situation can be ideal. Of course, on condition that they have someone to be dependent on. A wife's dependence on her husband, or vice versa, that's the norm: to stay together, not to stray too far, to think twice before every step. There's lots of legitimacy for intense togetherness.

From this description, it seems that what was "beneficial" was not the stress of war as such but the particular behaviors and expectations the Gulf War legitimized or fostered.

On the other hand, certain types of personalities were particularly stressed by the conditions of the war. According to Eli Chen, formerly chief psychologist of the IDF Medical Corps and currently head of Machom Ya'ad, "People characterized by control and activity have to wait passively now, and this is difficult for them." Chen also reports on a dependent patient who suffered intense feelings of abandonment when her live-in boyfriend left to spend the war with his widowed mother.

Some people sought help from the various hotlines. Most of the help sought was for specifically war-related stress, fear, and sleep disorders. According to the psychologists quoted, the Gulf War gave legitimacy to acknowledging and talking about such problems. That legitimization also brought to the hotlines some people with preexisting problems not related to the war.

Kroll's (1991) article also reports cases of first hospitalizations connected with the war, including people who obsessively sealed their entire apartments and people who blamed themselves for the war. It mentions a young man who attributed the war to his recent abandonment of religious observance and to a female soldier who felt so guilty for the war that she tried to kill herself.

Thus the article makes it plain that people responded to the war in a variety of ways, in keeping with their personalities and outlooks. Many long-term psychotherapy patients evidently managed well enough without their regular sessions; but some suffered from circumstances and pressures created by the war. Yet other people who had not previously been patients sought help, most on the hotlines for war-related difficulties, a few at hospitals for major problems in the psychotic symptom spectrum.

On the whole, the emphasis of Kroll's article is on the ability of most therapy patients to manage without their therapists during the war. Neither the writer nor any of the people quoted, however, suggest that there were any long-term improvements. The article raises, but does not answer, the question of how long the so-called beneficial effects lasted. Dr. Eli Chen predicted that they would be short term, with symptoms and other manifestations abating for a few weeks only to surface again with the war's end.

We now turn to observations on psychiatric, not merely psychotherapy, patients.

## Kaplan Hospital: The Saddam Syndrome

This report was written by a group of psychiatrists, Drs. Talmon, Guy, Mure, Rafes, and Naor (1992), on six patients who came urgently to the psychiatric emergency room of Kaplan Hospital in Rehovot, on the

periphery of the greater Tel Aviv area, during the first two weeks of the
Gulf War, between January 17 and 21, 1991.

The authors observe that during the war, a large number of patients
presented at the emergency rooms around the country, seeking help for
tension, irritability, discomfort, insomnia, and various autonomic and
even conversive reactions. In their view, some of the complaints can be
considered "normative adjustment reactions," while others are "acute
stress reactions" caused by the wartime threat. Their paper, published in
*HaRefuah (Medicine)*, the official journal of the Israeli Medical Association, focuses on six patients who "suffered from reactive psychotic episodes for the first time in their lives." In ordinary times, the authors
note, their hospital sees an average of only one such new psychiatric
patient without previous psychosis every two weeks. They attribute the
sixfold increase to the pressures of the war and term the "typical and
common symptoms along with delusional ideas . . . [in which] Saddam
[was] the only persecutor the "Saddam syndrome."

The following is a summary of the six cases they describe:

1. The first was a 66-year-old woman living alone who reached the
emergency room with signs of hyperventilation and in a state of hysteria.
At the first alarm she had gone into a panic, with generalized physical
discomfort and a feeling that she was swallowing her tongue. The day
before she sought help, she awoke in the middle of the night with a bad
stomachache, which she was convinced was caused by Saddam Hussein,
whom she saw standing in her bedroom. Terrified, she was sure there
had been a chemical attack, and in trying to inject herself with atropin,
the nerve-gas antidote distributed with the gas masks, accidently
squirted it in her face. In the emergency room, she expressed the conviction that the entire war was directed against her personally. She had no
other perceptual disturbances but displayed impaired judgment and
lack of self-perception. She refused both the medical and psychological
treatment offered and went home. A week later, she told a hospital
staffer who called that she felt much better.

2. The second case was a 30-year-old divorcee and mother of two
who was brought to the hospital by her family in a state of psychotic
paranoia that had begun with the first alarm. During that alarm, she
went into a panic accompanied by psychomotor paralysis and delusions
that the war was being fought against her personally and that gas was
seeping through cracks in the wall. She was brought to the hospital a
week later in a catatonic state and covered head to foot in clothing for
protection against chemicals. Crying and suspicious, she refused to let
go of her gas mask. She told the doctors that "Saddam attacked Israel
because of me."

3. The third case was a 33-year-old married businessman who was brought to the hospital in a state of extreme agitation after having become violent and broken things at home. In the emergency room, he grabbed a stethoscope from one of the doctors and began to examine the hospital walls. He demanded to speak immediately with the prime minister, the Lubavitcher Rebbe (an esteemed religious authority living in New York), and the IDF chief of staff, claiming that he had been contacted and given vital information that the country's water supply had been infected with viruses. Among the various auditory hallucinations he described were hallucinations of hearing alarms that had not in fact been sounded.

4. The fourth case was a 35-year-old father of two who reached the emergency room in a state of acute paranoia. Since the beginning of the war, he had severe sleep disturbances and felt strong tension and anxiety, with characteristic somatic symptoms. In the hospital, he spun lengthy and involved theories around the war. For example, he claimed that the missle strike in Ramat Gan had never happened but was merely a propaganda ploy by the Israeli government and media.

5. The fifth patient was a 77-year-old woman who still worked giving private English lessons. She was brought to the emergency room by her family in an acute psychotic state 10 days after the start of the war. Following the first alarm, when she panicked and ran out of her house, she developed persecutory, erotomanic, and sexual delusions and visual and auditory hallucinations.

6. The sixth patient was a 40-year-old mother of four, who up until then had been a competent housewife. She came to the emergency room the first week of the war on account of a severe anxiety reaction manifested in fears that she and her children would be poisoned by gas. In the hospital, she displayed regressive behavior, withdrawal, overdependence on her children, and temper tantrums. Examination showed overwhelming anxiety, affect frozen with fear, and persistent punitive thoughts of psychotic intensity of gas seeping into the house and killing the entire family.

The authors consider the Saddam syndrome a brief reactive psychosis. As they explain it, it differs from most other psychoses and resembles the transient psychotic reactions sometimes observed in combat soldiers. As stated above, none of these admissions had a history of prior psychosis. Two had predisposing vulnerability—one of them a neurological impairment, the other a history of school problems and a schizophrenic mother—but without the trigger of the Gulf War, the authors claim, their psychosis may never have erupted. None of the other four showed any clear etiological signs. At the nine-month follow-up, the two

with predisposing factors had not recovered. The other four recovered
rapidly and maintained their prewar adjustment levels.

## Shalvata Mental Health Center: Double Bookkeeping

In describing the wartime behavior of his schizophrenic patients at
the Shalvata Mental Health Center in Hod Hasharon, on the periphery
of the scudded area, Professor Levy (Levy A., 1991) applies the term
"double bookkeeping," coined by Bleuler (1950), to convey the capacity
of acute psychotics to simultaneously remain detached from and in contact with reality.

During the Gulf War, he observed, most of the patients were aware
that a war was in process and knew the major details. Some patients
listened to the radio constantly and notified the staff on hearing the
"nahash tzefa" alert. Many were unusually restless and paced the halls in
a manner that, in his view, resembled the nervous anticipatory behavior
of the general population. Most cooperated during alerts, went willingly
to the air-raid shelter, helped out with older or handicapped patients,
readily put on their gas masks, and were not frightened by the distorted
facades that the masks presented.

On the other hand, it was all but impossible to discuss the patients'
fears with them, either individually or in groups. For the most part, they
spoke about the situation in vague clichés, ignored the subject, or recounted their own problems over and over. Ventilation could not be
achieved. Moreover, some patients assimilated the war into their psychotic productions. One claimed that the war had not yet started; another
complained that he was being prevented from providing the authorities
with information crucial to winning it; yet another proclaimed there was
no need to worry, since the war was already over. Nor was cooperation
during alerts complete. Some patients were quite detached as they were
being led to the shelter. A few seemed totally unaware of what was
happening. For example, during one alert, as everyone was rushing to
the shelter, one woman sat frozen in front of the television with a distant
smile on her face, off in her own world.

## Beer Ya'acov Mental Health Center: Well-Disciplined Patients

The following observations of the psychiatric inpatients at the Beer
Ya'acov Mental Health Center (approximately 15 miles from Tel Aviv)
were written by the head of the hospital, Dr. Arie Schlosberg (unpublished manuscript) and appear in his general survey of the reactions
of Israeli civilians to the missile attacks. During the preparatory period

starting in December 1990, Dr. Schlosberg relates, the patients were briefed on the threat of war and chemical attack, practiced putting on their gas masks, and helped seal rooms. Then:

> During the war they were disciplined, even the long-standing schizophrenic patients. Some were anxious, others denied the situation (very few with psychotic denial—"Saddam is my brother," "there is no war for me—only for you"). There were signs of somatization and some regression. On the whole we were agreeably surprised to find that they reacted adequately, without any exacerbations of their illness. Some patients refused to put on their masks, some for valid reasons (difficulty in breathing), a few for psychotic reasons, and still others due to noncooperation owing to personality disorders. At the beginning of the war there were many postpsychotics who asked to be admitted for a short time; a few days later they were discharged, after being reassured.

## Beersheva Mental Health Center: No Change in Patients' Clinical State

Drs. Grisaru, Paronsky, Zabow, and Belmaker (1993) made observations of acute psychotics (30 schizophrenics and 5 manics) in the closed ward of a psychiatric hospital in the southern part of Israel. No missiles fell in the southern region, and once it became clear that the Scuds were trained on the center of the country, many individuals ignored the sirens. The hospital staff was obviously not free to do that.

The authors report that the large majority of patients cooperated with instructions, entered the sealed room during the alarms, and wore gas masks, but that a small number did not. They also report that there was no perceptible change in the patients' condition after the start of the war or after the sound of any given alarm, and they attribute this to the patients' self-absorption:

> After the first attack (when one patient remained outside the sealed room) every single patient entered the sealed room calmly during the subsequent strikes and remained there for from 15–240 minutes. In each episode about 2–4 patients in the sealed room refused to put on a gas mask, and the staff (as instructed) did not force them to. There were different patients who refused gas masks during each missile barrage, and there did not appear to be any correlation with clinical diagnosis or clinical state. Those patients with improving psychoses helped the staff with putting on the gas masks of the more psychotic patients. The staff, which numbered only 3–6 nurses and nurses' assistants on any single shift, did not report any psychotic exacerbations, agitation or panic attacks in the sealed room or as a result of wearing a gas mask. In fact, there were no noticeable changes in the patients' clinical state compared with the period before the missile attacks began or compared with the period before the air raid siren on the day of each attack. . . . In retrospect this does not seem surprising, since these patients are highly preoccupied with their internal world and concrete needs.

## Talbieh Mental Health Center: Holocaust Survivors

Drs. Robinson and Netanel (1991) conducted a study on Holocaust survivor psychiatric patients at the Talbieh Mental Health Center in Jerusalem.

They report that during the last week of the Gulf War, 13 of the psychiatric inpatients at this hospital were Holocaust survivors. Seven of them showed no reaction to the war. Of the remaining six, two had been admitted specifically because of their reaction to the Gulf War: an elderly woman with no previous psychiatric hospitalization who reacted with deep anxiety, and another woman with a history of manic-depression, who was readmitted an account of anxiety and deep depression. Of the other four, one was an elderly survivor who became more suspicious of his wife and was violent toward her; two who became frightened and tense whenever a siren sounded; and one, a chronic schizophrenic hospitalized for many years, who became convinced that the doctors had injected gas into her room and that she had heard Saddam Hussein proclaiming that there was no war and that it was merely propaganda spread by the former Israeli prime minister, Menachem Begin.

In the outpatient clinic, there were 18 Holocaust survivors during the Gulf War. Only four of them showed reactions to the war. Their symptoms included anxiety, revival of Holocaust memories, fear of hunger, deepened depression, concentration difficulties, sleep disturbances, tension, and psychosomatic complaints.

These findings are difficult to analyze because of the limited information given and because the authors neither make nor exclude any association between the patients' illnesses and their Holocaust experience. The sparse description, however, suggests that the Holocaust-survivor psychiatric inpatients were not much different from non-Holocaust psychiatric patients. The inpatients seem to divide into those who were oblivious of the war and those who reacted to it either with exacerbation of a previous disorder or with a newly developed disorder whose anxiety-laden or delusional contents were related to the Gulf War. This division is similar to that of the psychiatric patients described in the empirical studies discussed below.

Among the outpatients, the picture is even less clear. At least some of the four whose symptoms are mentioned seem to have suffered a reactivation of Holocaust traumas, in that their "reactions to the Gulf War" included the revival of Holocaust memories and other posttrauma symptoms.

The clinical impressions presented above suggest that most of the mentally ill responded adequately to the exigencies of the war and were sufficiently in touch with reality to be aware that a war was in progress and to comply with the safety instructions. Only a few failed to put on their gas masks and go peacefully to the sealed room. While some of the patients incorporated the war into their psychotic productions, none of the reports, with the possible exception of that on the Holocaust-survivor patients in Jerusalem, points to psychotic exacerbation. Nor are there any complaints of having insufficient staff or preparations to handle the emergency.

How generalizable are these impressions? Are they supported by systematic empirical research? For a fuller answer, we turn to the more organized and systematic studies carried out by several hospitals in Israel on their psychiatric patients during and shortly after the Gulf War.

## Abarbanel Mental Health Center

This study was conducted in Abarbanel Mental Health Center, which is the largest psychiatric hospital in Israel, with hundreds of inpatients. The hospital is located in Bat Yam, within the greater Tel Aviv region. There were several missile strikes in its vicinity early in the war, and residents in the area reported, hearing rattling windows and the loud boom of the landings. The study was carried out by the psychiatrist, Dr. Yuval Melamed; the hospital director, Professor Avner Elizur, Dr. Henry Schur, and myself (in preparation).

It is a retrospective study of 95 patients with various degrees of disturbances. Three groups of patients were examined: 33 acute schizophrenics in a closed ward; 24 chronic schizophrenics in an open rehabilitation ward; and 38 chronic schizophrenic outpatients. The study was conducted a short time after the war. Patients were asked to assess themselves at three points in time—before, during, and after the war—by rating themselves on a scale of 1 (poor) to 5 (good) on 12 different dimensions of functioning and symptomatology, such as social functioning, somatic problems, concern for others, restlessness, and grooming.

In the acute group, average scores on these 12 dimensions improved slightly during the war and continued to improve afterward. In particular these patients registered improvements in social functioning, vocational functions, withdrawal, and grooming. There was no indication of regression or detrioration in this group, and the patients' self-reports were confirmed by the impressions of the hospital staff. However, the chronic patients, both outpatients and those in the rehabilitation ward, reported a slight deterioration during the war (in social functioning, work functioning, and grooming), followed by a return to baseline afterward. Yet they also showed improvement in some areas, such as concern for self and greater interest in external events. In fact, most of the patients read newspapers and watched television during the war. Unfortunately, once the war was over, things went back to "normal," and their interest in their surroundings waned.

The patients' emotional response to the war can be considered appropriate. All three groups reported increased disquiet during the war as well as a drop in mood; no patients were described as manic. Their emotional response is similar to that of the Shalvata patients described by Professor Amihay Levy. One implication of these findings is that whatever improvement in functioning there was occurred *despite* the increased sense of tension, which had to be overcome.

Another way of examining whether or not there was a deterioration in the patients' condition was to look at changes in their consumption of medication during the war. In general, there was no need to increase medication in any of the groups during the war: acute patients' dosages were gradually lowered (as is usually the case), and chronic patients' dosages remained stable. Interestingly, some of the chronic outpatients reported that they reduced the intake of tranquilizers on their own so as not to sleep through an alert.

The authors attribute the difference in the response of the acute and chronic patients to several factors. One is the different level of support the two groups received. The closed wards in which the acute patients stayed provided them with structure and protection unavailable to the outpatients and with a higher patient–staff ratio. Moreover, the families of acute patients tended to visit more and to be more supportive than those of chronic patients. The second reason is the difference in the impairment of the two groups. According to the authors, the acute patients are essentially less severely impaired than the chronic ones, so the extreme external stress of the war suppressed their psychotic manifestations. Finally, the improvement of the acute patients is in keeping with the natural course of their illness, where the acute phase is generally followed by amelioration or remission of the disorder. Whatever the reason, it seems that the war did not affect the acute patients adversely or impede their recovery.

In summary, most of the findings of this study seem to favor the contention that collective external stress has little if any effect on mental patients. The authors suggest that the demands of the war may have helped some of the acute patients: that is, forcing them to attend to reality and distracting them from their inner chaos led to a higher level of inner organization and improved functioning. But it is also possible to interpret the data as indicating that the acute patients were fairly oblivious to the war and were getting better in any event. As for the slight deterioration of the chronic patients, while this may indicate that external stress can lead to regression in chronic mental patients, it should be remembered that even the chronic patients showed improvement in some areas and that their deterioration was mild and transient.

## Pardessia Medical Mental Health Center

This is a three-part study by Marc Gelkopf with Drs. Aviv Bendor and Mircea Sigal (Bendor, Gelkopf, & Sigal, 1993; Bendor, Sigal, & Gelkopf, 1994; Gelkopf, Ben-Dor, & Sigal, unpublished manuscript).

The study was conducted in a 300-bed psychiatric hospital in the central region of Israel between the fifth and the eighth day of the war. The researchers examined a large sample of 250 inpatients from three groups, all of whom were diagnosed according to DSM-III-R criteria: (1) 167 long-term patients, mostly hospitalized for over 10 years with *schizophrenia, residual type* (that is, chronic schizophrenics); (2) 46 *active phase schizophrenics* (that is, people recently hospitalized in the midst of an acute episode), most of whom were admitted for limited periods of time, then returned to their homes and occupations; and (3) 37 *residual phase* schizophrenics, who, like the active schizophrenics, had been recently hospitalized for an acute episode but whose illness was in remission or responding to treatment.

The researchers composed two questionnaires on the patients' cognitions, emotions, and behavior during the alarms. One consisted of 11 questions answered by the patients during the morning meetings; the other contained 5 questions for the staff, who reported their observations on the conduct of each of the patients present in the hospital during the alarms. Changes in treatment during the war were also examined.

In the *cognitive* realm, only 70% of the patients stated that they were aware that a war was in progress, with no significant group differences, and the majority understood that the country was being bombarded. That is, close to a third of the patients, whether chronic, acute, or recovering schizophrenics, claimed total ignorance of the war.

Similarly, a certain proportion of the patients in each group reported not hearing the alarms. However, here there were significant group differences, with only 64% of the acute patients reporting having heard the previous alarm as opposed to 83% of the chronic patients and 90% of those in the residual phase. The authors suggest that the difference might be accounted for by the possibility that patients in the active phase of their illness were more likely to have integrated the alarms into their paranoid systems and were more preoccupied with their hallucinations than chronic or recovering patients, who are less prone to psychotic elaboration.

The *emotional* responses of the patients in the active and nonactive phases of their illness were also different. To the question of whether they felt anxious, secure, or apathetic when they wore their masks, the acute schizophrenics were the most likely to report feeling secure or apathetic and the least likely to report feeling anxiety. Only 3.8% of them admitted to anxiety, as opposed to around 25% of the chronic patients and about 40% of those in remission. Over half of them reported feeling nothing, in contrast to around a third of the patients in each of the other two groups. Moreover, proportionally fewer of the acute schizophrenics reported feeling worried during the alarms. Only about half of them acknowledged worrying about themselves, as opposed to three-quarters of the patients in the other two groups. Conversely, those in the residual phase were the most likely to express worry about friends and family.

The staff also distinguished between the acute schizophrenics and the others. They viewed the chronic patients as least likely to be anxious and the acute patients as displaying a combination of detachment and panic. According to staff reports, a higher proportion of the acute than the other patients showed more apathy than usual, and a higher proportion of them showed panic, though the rates of panic were low in all groups.

With regard to *behavior*, the staff reported that most of the patients in all the groups were well disciplined during the alarms, obeyed staff instructions, and put on their masks. Only about 10% of the patients on average had to be pressured to enter the sealed room and don their masks. There was also relatively little erratic behavior, and most of that was among the acute patients.

In their discussion, the authors emphasize that most of the patients were not only aware of the threat but also quite frightened for both themselves and their families, and differed primarily in how they coped with their concerns. The patients' coping, they point out, ran from a combination of overt denial and overt indications of anxiety among the acute patients to normal anxiety symptoms among the residual-phase patients.

The researchers also examined the patients' charts and compared the *changes in treatment* that were instituted during the war with those initiated in similar groups of patients during the same period the year before. Five types of treatment change were examined: prescription of new medication; increase in dosage; totally new treatment; transfer from an open to a closed ward; and use of physical restraint.

Comparison showed that both active-phase (acute) and residual-phase (acute in remission) schizophrenics underwent more treatment changes during the war than comparable groups in the same time period the year before, but residual-type chronic patients did not. Among the acute schizophrenics, rates of all five treatment changes were higher: 34% received new medication as opposed to 13% the year before; 43% as opposed to 18% had their dosages increased; 43% as opposed to 24% received a totally new treatment; and 23% in contrast to only 5% the year previous were held in restraint. More residual-phase patients (acute in remission) also received new medication and a totally new type of treatment than the year before. The authors admit that some of the changes may have stemmed not only from the patients' behavior but also from the anxiety of the staff that they might have to cope with violent or uncooperative patients during an attack.

## Shalvata Mental Health Center: Responses to the Threat of War

Like Dr. Amihay Levy's clinical observations reported above, this study was carried out on the psychiatric inpatients at Shalvata Mental Health Center in Hod Hasharon, on the periphery of the central region. Conducted by Drs. Levin, Barkai, Levkowitch, Weiser, Levy, and Nuemann (unpublished manuscript), this study examined the response of psychiatric patients not to the war itself but to the *threat* of the war. Their rationale was that acknowledgment of the threat would help people cope with the danger, whereas denial would hamper coping.

More precisely, the study compared the answers of 10 schizophrenic inpatients in a closed ward to self-report questionnaires with those of 16 staff members one week prior to the Coalition attack. The subjects were asked to rate the likelihood of war on a scale of 0 (certain that war will not break out) to 10 (certain that it will) and to fill out Spielberger's inventories of state and trait anxiety, anger, and curiosity.

Patients' assessments of the likelihood of war were lower than those of staff. In the authors' view, this suggests that the patients tended to deny the danger of war, possibly on account of the intense self-involvement implicit in their psychosis. This interpretation is consistent with Dr. Levy's observation that during the war the patients were unwilling to discuss the war or deal with it on a verbal level even though they clearly knew that a war was going on. It is also consistent with the view of the Pardessia study authors that the patients in that hospital tended to deny the dangers they felt.

Patients had higher trait anxiety than staff, but similar levels of state anxiety. The authors conclude that trait anxiety is associated with mental health, while state anxiety reflects the magnitude of the external threat. The finding also points to an underlying awareness of the threat, such as was found in the Pardessia study, despite its denial on a cognitive level.

Patients had higher levels of state anger than staff. According to the authors, this may reflect either the patients' response to the threat of war or their feelings at being locked up in a closed ward.

The authors also examined the subjects' trait anger and state and trait curiosity. They found that these were not significantly different in the patients and staff. The authors make no attempt to account for the similarity. The finding does, however, reinforce observations made in other reports that many patients showed an interest in the events of the war and even followed them on television.

## CONCLUSIONS

The overall findings from both organized studies and clinical observations at various hospitals and mental health agencies throughout the country show a clear and fairly consistent pattern:

1. *Acute schizophrenics* tended to be fairly oblivious to the war [Abarbanel, Beersheva], though it colored the content of the delusions or hallucinations of some of them [Beer Yalakov, Shalvata, Pardessia]. At Pardessia, the staff viewed most of the acute schizophrenics as detached, and some of the patients there reported that they felt nothing when they wore their gas masks. At the same time, the behavior of the acute schizophrenic was for the most part compliant, and only a few succumbed to panic or engaged in erratic conduct.

Two of the reports observed that these patients functioned on two levels at the same time. Dr. Levy at Salvata described their "double bookkeeping," whereby most of the patients were aware that a war was going on, complied with the emergency instructions, and exhibited nervous behavior in keeping with the threat, but at the same time refused to talk about it. Dr. Gelkopf and colleagues at Pardessia described cognitive awareness, on the one hand, and what they considered feigned indifference, on the other. In short, these patients were seen to have been aware yet unaware, agitated yet indifferent, compliant yet detached.

Findings differed on the need for changes in treatment because of the war, however. At Abarbanel, acute patients' medication was not altered. At Pardessia, treatment was changed considerably for the acute patients, somewhat less for the acute patients in the process of recovery, and not at all for the chronic patients. The researchers acknowledge that some of the changes may have stemmed primarily from the staff's anxiety over the possibility of having to deal with violent behavior during an actual missile attack rather than from the patients' needs or changes in behavior. The difference in the two hospitals underscores the important role that the staff of mental health institutions play in acute patients' conduct during times of stress.

2. *Schizophrenics not actively delusional* (chronics, acutes in remission) apparently became more reality oriented and socially concerned for the duration of the war. This was reflected in their helpfulness and cooperation with others, in their interest in the radio and newspapers, and in an appropriate increase in tension [Abarbanel, Shalvata]. There was agreement across hospitals that there was no need to change treatment or increase medication in chronic patients on account of any exacerbation of problems. In fact, some outpatients actually reduced their medication on their own to ensure that they would wake up for the alerts [Abarbanel].

3. In a very small number of *cases with no prior history of psychosis,* the stress of the war may have caused a brief transient psychosis or triggered a first episode of more enduring psychosis in those with some kind of constitutional (neurological, psychological) vulnerability.

These conclusions should all be tempered, however, by the preliminary and somewhat tentative nature of the studies and observations on which they are based. As pointed out throughout this book, conducting research during wartime is a formidable undertaking. Studying psychiatric patients is even more so.

Given the cognitive distortions inherent in most psychiatric disorders, the self-reports of psychiatic patients, which were either the basis or the major component of all the empirical studies reviewed here, must be accepted cautiously. The retrospective reporting required of the patients in the Abarbanel study raises all the questions of retrospective reporting in general and plenty more in this case.

Nor do parallel staff reports necessarily provide an adequate standard of comparison. While unofficial staff observations tallied with the self-reports of the acute and chronic patients at Abarbanel, at Pardessia staff and patients did not always share the same views. There the staff rated 80% in all three groups examined as not being anxious at all or only somewhat anxious, in contrast to only about 30% of the patients who claimed not to be worried either about themselves or relatives. The authors favor the patients' view. They attribute the discrepancy to the staff's having been impressed by the patients' disciplined behavior during the alarms and to the fact that the dangers of the missiles and their weighty responsibilities during the alerts did not leave them much time to check the patients' states of mind.

Nonetheless, the studies and observations reviewed here provide some support for each of the three predictions presented at the start of the chapter. Psychosis was seen to be caused or triggered by the stress of war in a small number of people with no prior history of psychosis. Acute schizophrenics were mostly seen to be oblivious to and unaffected by the war, and chronic schizophrenics showed some improvement.

# 9

# Soldiers in Restraint

In contrast to every other war in which Israel has been involved, in the Gulf War Israel Defense Forces (IDF) soldiers were not engaged in combat. Although the country was subjected to 39 missile attacks that killed two, injured others, and caused extensive damage to property, the army was kept on a leash. It could do nothing to prevent, mitigate, or punish the attacks in which enemy weapons were trained on Israel's civilian population. This is a disconcerting situation for any army and all the more so for the IDF.

Emotionally, the restraint struck a dissonant chord, not only because the natural instinct to strike back when hit was kept in check, but also because it contrasted so sharply with the image and self-concept that the IDF had built up over the years and that Israelis—soldiers and civilians alike—had internalized. The image, supported by the army's performance in previous crises, was of an assertive defense force that responded in an organized, swift, and unambiguous manner to enemy aggression. It was the force (both the power and the body) that maintained the nation's sovereignty and protected the lives of its citizens. It was conceived before the State of Israel was officially established and grew up with the State, against the memory of the Holocaust and the victimization to which Jews were subjected before they had an army. So in addition to the serving as the mighty sling of David that foiled Israel's enemies, the IDF was also seen—and saw itself—as a kind of raised fist ensuring that such a history of helpless victimization would never again be repeated.

The policy of restraint in the Gulf War was carried out against this special Israeli sense of what its army was and how it should conduct itself. From a certain perspective, the IDF's strength and the country's faith in that strength are what made that restraint possible. Had there been doubts as to the army's capacity to come to the country's defense more actively, were that deemed necessary, the pressure for action might have been greater, if only as a proof of strength, and the wait-and-see position less tenable. (There were people, however, who argued that the IDF's restraint might cause the Arabs to think it was weak.) Nonetheless, the enforced passivity did not sit well with the deeply internalized image of an assertive defense force protecting family and country. Nor could it help but echo individual and collective memories of what had happened in the past when Jews were not able to take up arms in their own defense.

On a more mundane level, the soldiers who were called on to serve during this period had to contend with immediate, practical stressors. Many of them were young men and women doing their two or three years of compulsory army service, as required by Israeli law. Others were somewhat older reserve soldiers who had completed their regular service and were now called up posthaste to emergency duty. Yet others were in the regular army, their hours extended and leaves canceled. Because of the overhanging threat, there was a sense of urgency to their duty. But for many of them the content of that duty was not entirely clear. Peacetime routines were in abeyance, but wartime routines had not been adapted in all units. Especially at the beginning, soldiers in some units arrived at their posts, then didn't know what to do there. Nor did their commanders. Even where matters were less confusing, however, many of the soldiers were there to be on hand, "just in case." In other words, they had a lot of waiting to do. In practical terms, this is what the policy of restraint translated into for many soldiers: being poised for a battle that they had no way of knowing would actually take place, or when, and enduring the tedium and tension inherent in the interim.

To make matters worse, while the soldiers were poised for action, their families were virtually sitting ducks at home, and they could do nothing to aid or comfort them. In actuality, soldiers faced much the same danger as civilians. Yet they had the added burden of being separated from and unable to protect the families they felt responsible for, both personally and as IDF soldiers, with all that meant.

The IDF, all too experienced in preparing soldiers for battle, never before had to consider how soldiers "on hold" would cope while the people they were supposed to protect sustained one missile attack after another. The IDF had little to go on either to predict soldiers' responses or to know how best to help soldiers withstand the special rigors of such a situation. The one indication that came from the mental health profession portended badly. It was based on the widely accepted view of the Israeli man as action oriented and impatient (Lazarus, 1986; Lieblich, 1983). In 1974, at a conference on stress sponsored by Tel Aviv University, the prominent stress researcher Richard Lazarus referred to a sense of mastery as the typical coping method employed by Israelis (Lazarus, 1986). He defined Israelis as having an internal locus of control style (following Parson & Schneider, 1974), being convinced that they are able to shape their own fate. The coping ego ideal that has been emerging among the Israelis, claimed Lazarus, is an active one, involving aggressive striving toward autonomy and control of external events, as opposed to the passive mastery that seeks to manage the sources of one's security by self-control and by inhibition of aggression. Based on these assertions, one may have predicted that in the Gulf War, in which Israeli soldiers had only limited opportunities to use direct active coping, emotional difficulties would arise.

That is quite far from what happened. This chapter presents the findings of five separate studies conducted by the Israeli army, air force, and navy, aimed at assessing the extent and nature of distress among soldiers during the Gulf War. The studies focus primarily on soldiers in the central region, the area at highest risk for Scud missile attacks. The first three studies examine the general population of soldiers. The last two studies focus on soldiers who applied to army mental health clinics during the Gulf War.

## STUDY 1: ISRAELI AIR FORCE

In the first weeks of the war, the psychology branch of the Israeli air force carried out a study of the coping of air force personnel in the central region. The study, conducted by Orit Luria (1991), assessed 308 officers and regular soldiers from 12 units. Forty percent of subjects were male; 86.6% were single; and 42.7% resided in or around an area that was hit by missiles. Most had professional or service rather than combat assignments (for example, medical, intelligence, communications). The survey had three major aims: (1) to identify the war's major stressors; (2) to identify the characteristic expressions of the stress; and (3) to identify the ways in which the soldiers coped with the stresses.

### Major Stressors

Subjects were asked to rate the stressfulness of 12 events or features of the Gulf War (such as false air-raid sirens or being alone during an alert) on a 5-point scale ranging from "hardly stressful to all" to "extremely stressful." Findings showed that the main stressor was the fear that a family member would be hurt. Sixty-eight percent of the subjects ranked this as very or extremely stressful. No other stressor was reported to be so disturbing by such a high proportion of the subjects. The second most common stressor was "uncertainty, not knowing what's going to happen next," but it was endorsed far less often, by only 39.6% of subjects.

Further analyses showed that the assessment of stressors was affected by gender and proximity to the strikes. Women soldiers generally assigned higher stress ratings to the various war events than men, analogous to the gender differences observed among civilians in Chapter 4. Similarly, soldiers whose families resided in or near an area hit by missles tended to rate the various events as more stressful than subjects whose families spent the war elsewhere.

**Stress Effects**

Four different types of stress effects were examined: somatic, emotional, cognitive, and behavioral. Subjects were asked to indicate on a 5-point scale ranging from "not at all," to "very high" the extent to which their stress was manifested in each of these areas. High or very high levels of *emotional* stress effects (in the form of fear, apprehension, depression, or restlessness) were reported by 18.2% of subjects and a moderate amount by a further 31.9%. High or very high levels of *behavioral* stress effects, primarily disordered eating (overeating or undereating), sleep difficulties (lack of sleep or oversleeping), low frustration tolerance (nervousness, outbursts of temper), and changes in activity level (hyperactivity or apathy/withdrawal), were reported by 19.9% of subjects, with another 20.9% reporting a moderate amount. *Somatic* effects were less common. Ten percent of the air force personnel in this study reported a high degree of somatic stress effects, and another 17.6% reported a moderate amount. The most common somatic effects were trembling, stomachaches, diarrhea, and headaches. Finally, only 7% of soldiers in this study reported a high degree of *cognitive* impairment during the war. A further 15.8% reported a moderate amount of cognitive disturbances, in the form of concentration difficulties, forgetfulness, and the need to invest a great deal of energy to carry out simple tasks.

As with the stress ratings, there were also gender differences in the severity of stress responses, with women tending to report higher stress effects than men in each of the above areas except for cognition. On the other hand, there was no difference in the types of stress effects reported by those who lived close to the areas of the missile attacks and those who lived farther away. In both cases, stress effects were primarily in the emotional and behavioral domains.

## Coping

Subjects were also asked to rate the helpfulness of 19 different coping behaviors or resources during the war on a 5-point scale from "hardly helpful at all" to "extremely helpful." Fifty to 67.5% of the respondents rated the following coping resources as very or extremely helpful (in descending order): being with others, faith in the protective devices, faith in the state and the IDF, ties with family members, ties with friends, maintaining normal routines, and communications media. These resources are largely ideological and social. A smaller but still significant portion of the respondents (30–42%) reported that they found the sense of participating as a soldier in the war effort, concern for someone else (child, pet), and humor either very or extremely help-ful. However, only 15.4% of the air force soldiers queried felt that their commander had helped them significantly in coping with the stresses of the war, while 57% reported that their commander was of little assis-tance.

On the whole, the responses of men and women were similar, though more women tended to regard social support (friends, family, commanders) as helpful than did men.

Luria (1991) concludes her study with the finding that although about half the respondents reported feeling at least a moderate amount of war-related stress, 70% of those queried felt that they were able to cope with it either well or very well. We may observe that this figure corre-sponds roughly to the percentage that reported having experienced no more than moderate stress effects in any of the areas investigated. It also corresponds with the findings of the Israeli Institute of Applied Social Research (Chapter 2) that 70% of the general public of Tel Aviv and Haifa reported that they were adjusting well to the war and with the finding of the IDF Department of Behavioral Sciences survey (Chapter 2) that 73% of those they queried in the second week of the war reported that they were coping well or very well. In other words, soldiers' sense of mastery was much the same as that of the rest of the population.

## STUDY 2: ISRAELI NAVY

The Israeli navy conducted a study of its logistic and support per-sonnel at a base in the central region during the Gulf War. The study, carried out by Gil Esroni (1991), examined the soldiers' unit and personal morale; manifestations of tension; and the conviction that they, their families, and the civilian population as a whole could protect themselves. The study also explored soldiers' use of time, their sense of being informed, and the interpersonal relationships within the unit. It was conducted on 158 subjects in January 1991. About half the sample were officers; about half were female.

The questionnaires were administered about a week into the war, most of them on January 21 and 22, before the Scuds had caused any major damage. But 45 were administered on January 23, the morning after a missile strike in Ramat Gan injured scores of people and totally destroyed eight apartment buildings. This accidental difference enables us to obtain not only a general sense of the impact of the war and its associated stresses on the soldiers but also a more specific sense of the direct impact of the major war event, the Scud attacks.

*Morale* was quite middling before the first major Scud strike and considerably lower on the morning after it. Before the strike, about half the soldiers rated their unit and personal moral as either high or very high (51% and 48%, respectively). After the strike, the proportion went down to about a third (34% and 33%, respectively).

Concomitantly, *manifestations of tension* increased considerably following the attack. Before that crucial date, 27% reported having considerable or a great deal of difficulty falling asleep; the day after, 44% told of such difficulties. Before, 35% reported strong or very strong feelings of uneasiness; the day after, the figure jumped to 56%. Before, only 9% reported a large or very large lack of appetite; the day after, 20% did.

The differences in the pre- and poststrike figures for morale and tension (1) suggest that the soldiers were affected by the same stressors as the civilian population, (2) show how labile and affected by the war events their mood was, and (3) coincide with the findings of a surge in anxiety among the civilian population following the missile attacks (see Chapter 2).

The soldiers' *beliefs about their own and others' safety,* however, remained fairly stable. What stands out in the set of questions pertaining to this subject is the evident difference in the soldiers' evaluation of their own and the army's capacity for self-defense, on the one hand, and that of the civilian population in general and of their families in particular, on the other hand.

Virtually all respondents (98%) stated that they knew what to do to protect themselves in the event of attack, and approximately three-quarters (78%) stated that they felt confident in their ability to do what was required. A similar percentage (77%) stated that they had faith in the army's defensive capacity. In contrast, fewer than half the respondents, 44%, believed that the civilian sector could protect itself in the event of an attack, and accordingly, only 52% felt that their immediate family would be able to do so.

The contrast reflects the reversal of home and front in the Gulf War, where soldiers were safe far from the battlefield while civilians on the "home front" were the targets of attack. The differences in assessments can actually be considered quite subjective. Aside from having better-fitting gas masks than the civilian population, soldiers and civilians were in much the same predicament vis-à-vis the enemy. Being in the center of Israel, these soldiers were no less at risk. It is merely a matter of chance that the Scuds happened to hit a residential area of Ramat Gan rather than, for example, the large military installation located only a few miles away. The contrast gives a better indication of the soldiers' emotional situation than of their objective one. Reinforcing the findings of the air force study, the findings of the navy study point to the soldiers' worry about their families being abandoned to fend for themselves. These findings also reinforce the suggestions of that study that the army framework (ideology, the sense of togetherness, and the sense of purpose) served as a major coping resource.

The generally middling morale (neither high nor notably low for most soldiers) and the manifestation of tension among a certain proportion of them may be considered in the context of three of the other measures.

*Interpersonal relations* in the unit were rated as good or very good by an average of 88% of the participants, with the after-strike ratings slightly better than the before-strike ones.

The soldiers' *sense of being informed* was also high, with 91% of the respondents viewing themselves as well informed about the war. Two-thirds stated that their commanders held group discussions about the situation. Anxiety levels were found to be higher among those whose commanders had not conducted such group talks.

On the other hand, the soldiers were generally less pleased with their *use of time*. Only 15% felt that their time was put to good use, with another 39% feeling that it was used reasonably well. Almost half (45%), however, judged that it was used poorly or very badly. As for exactly how the time was apportioned, it turns out that well over half was given over to waiting and emergency-related activities or to "make-work" such as washing floors, while only a bit over 40% was spent in work that could be seen as soldierly and useful, whether routine, nonwartime tasks or participation in operational problem-solving teams.

Differences were found for both rank and gender.

*Rank*

Officers reported high or very high unit and personal morale more often than ordinary soldiers (50% versus 35% and 54% versus 28%, respectively). And fewer of them reported difficulty in falling asleep (53% versus 83%) and loss of appetite (37% versus 51%). They made the same assessments as other soldiers, however, of their own, the public's, and their family's ability to protect themselves, and they felt neither better nor worse informed than other soldiers.

*Gender*

Men reported high levels of unit morale and personal morale more often than women (59% versus 27% and 57% versus 26%, respectively). They were also more likely than women to express faith in the ability of the civilian sector to protect itself (54% versus 34%). By the same token, women were more likely than men to report signs of tension, such as difficulty falling asleep (49% versus 13%), uneasiness (54% versus 29%), and loss of appetite (18% versus 8%).

## STUDY 3: SOLDIERS IN THE CENTRAL REGION

The most comprehensive of the three studies was conducted by the Mental Health Department of the IDF Medical Corps (Solomon, Margalit, Waysman, & Bleich, 1991) as part of an assessment of soldiers' mental health needs. It was a controlled study carried out on 659 soldiers in eight different army settings during the last week of January and in the first part of February 1991. Six of the eight groups consisted of soldiers serving on a variety of military installations throughout the central region. The other two were control groups: one consisting of soldiers who were outpatients at the IDF Central Mental Health Clinic, the other consisting of career officers who were assessed when they reported for routine army medical checkups.

The majority of subjects were single (from 67% to 96% in each group). Seventy-five percent were male, and 16% were officers. Regular soldiers (age 19–21) outnumbered both career and reserve soldiers in each of the groups, but there were more reservists in the patient group than in any of the others. The study assessed the soldiers' level of distress, their clinical picture, the correlates of their distress, and differences between the patients and nonpatients that might have borne on the one seeking help while the other did not.

## Levels of Distress

The soldiers' level of stress was measured in terms of their specifically stress-related sympotmatology, general symptomatology, and need for treatment.

Stress symptoms were tapped by a 20-item checklist of psychological and somatic symptoms characteristic of stress responses (for example, sleep difficulties, increased sensitivity to noise, hypervigilance, psychic numbing). The checklist was constructed by the research team on the basis of DSM-III-R criteria for posttraumatic stress disorder (PTSD) (APA, 1987). Although none of the subjects could qualify as posttraumatic for the simple reason that the diagnosis requires that the symptoms endure for at least a month, it was thought that the symptoms that make up the PTSD could serve to gauge the stress that people experience as they live through a potentially traumatic situation, and not only afterward. Participants were asked to rate their reactions on a scale ranging from 1 (never had symptom) to 4 (have symptom frequently). Their responses indicate a low to moderate level of stress-related distress, with the average symptom scores in the eight groups ranging from 1.6 to 2.5, the latter being the score in the patient group.

General psychiatric symptomatology was assessed by the Global Severity Index (GSI) of the Symptom Checklist 90 (SCL-90-R; Derogatis, 1977), a standardized measure with established psychometric properties that has been widely used in research in Israel and elsewhere. Subjects were asked to indicate the frequency with which they experienced each symptom on the list on a scale ranging from 1 (never) to 5 (frequently). The study calculated the percentage of subjects in each group whose levels of psychiatric symptomatology exceeded the norm for outpatients. This provides a rough indication of how many of them experienced a very high level of distress. It was found that though half of those in the patient group exceeded the outpatient norm, the rate was much lower in the other groups, where it ranged from 0% to 14%.

Need for treatment was assessed by a single yes–no item inquiring whether the respondent currently felt the need for psychological assistance. Only 4% of the subjects in the nonpatient group answered yes, and not a single officer did. Oddly, only 60% of the patient group answered in the affirmative.

## The Symptoms Picture

The endorsement of stress-related symptoms on the 20-item checklist was used to draw up a symptoms picture. The two most frequently endorsed symptoms, by both the patient and nonpatient groups, were increased sensitivity to noise, endorsed by 75% of the nonpatients and 74% of the patients, and hypervigilance, endorsed by 73% of the patients and a still high 55% of the nonpatients. It can be argued that these symptoms were functional in that they promote alertness, which was precisely what was called for in the Gulf War. The remaining 18 symptoms were endorsed, but by far fewer patients and nonpatients alike.

The findings on the level of distress and the symptoms picture refute both the expectation (discussed in Chapter 2) that during major catastrophes there would be widespread panic, and, conversely, the sanguine view that disasters do not heighten or induce emotional problems. The findings suggest that the truth lies somewhere in between. A significant proportion of the population surveyed in the current study reported some signs of stress-related tension, especially hypervigilance and increased sensitivity to noise. Moreover, the findings of the SCL-90-R show that a certain percentage of the soldiers suffered a high level of psychiatric symptomatology, and there were soldiers who either sought or felt the need for treatment. On the other hand, the overall percentage of soldiers who exceeded outpatient norms on the SCL-90-R was relatively low, the army's psychiatric services were far from swamped, and only 4% of the nonpatients felt sufficient distress to assert the need for treatment. This picture is consistent with that of the general population discussed in Chapter 2.

## Correlates of Distress

The second part of the study explored the connection between the soldiers' levels of distress (measured by the 20-item questionnaire and the SCL-90-R) and three moderating variables: sense of safety, social support, and coping style. All three were found to have a bearing on how much distress soldiers reported. Soldiers who gauged the danger to themselves and their families to be greater, who assessed their ability to cope in the event of chemical and conventional attack as lower, and who expressed little trust in the military authorities registered higher levels of distress than soldiers who felt safer. Soldiers who perceived a low level of support from the social network, particularly from commanding officers, also registered higher levels of distress. On the other hand, the more soldiers used problem-focused coping and distraction to cope with the stresses of the war, the less severe their distress. That is, soldiers who did their work or found work to do, and who read newspapers, talked to friends, or engaged in other occupations, reported lower levels of distress than soldiers who turned inward and mulled on the situation. This pattern of correlations was similar in all the study groups.

The role of each of these factors in moderating the response to extreme stress has been demonstrated in the past. High levels of perceived danger have been found to be associated with increased levels of distress among such diverse groups as combat soldiers (Solomon, Mikulincer, & Benbenishty, 1989b) and people in the vicinity of the Three Mile Island nuclear accident (Bromet, Schulberg, & Dunn, 1982). The ability of perceived self-efficacy to mitigate or prevent symptomatology was also shown in studies of combat soldiers, which found that the soldiers who possessed that sense of competence had lower rates of both acute combat stress reaction and chronic posttraumatic stress disorder than their companions-in-arms who were less confident of their ability to cope (Solomon, Weisenberg, Schwarzwald, & Mikulincer, 1988).

There is reason to believe that perceived threat and perceived self-efficacy work in tandem. According to Bandura (1977, 1982), whose work on perceived self-efficacy has laid the foundation for an extensive body of research, people constantly assess their capabilities, and these assessments guide their behavior. While people are ready to invest effort in activities that they deem within their powers and even to persevere in the face of obstacles, they tend to reduce the effort they put into tasks they consider beyond them, and to perform those tasks less effectively or to avoid the challenge altogether. Applied to Israel's soldiers in the Gulf War, the theory suggests that those who showed high levels of symptomatology put less effort into coping because they did not believe they could. It may well be that whether or not symptoms developed was a combined function of the soldiers' assessment of their own coping skills (perceived self-efficacy) and their perception of the degree of external threat (Lazarus & Folkman, 1984).

This general line of thinking is supported by the finding that active coping was associated with lower symptomatology. It seems that Israelis' preference for active coping notwithstanding, such coping apparently has advantages even in situations where action can do little to alleviate the threat.

Prior investigations have also demonstrated that supportive ties with others may mitigate the noxious effects of stress. Previous research by the IDF mental health branch (Solomon, Mikulincer, & Hobfoll, 1987) found that support from officers was especially effective in preventing acute combat stress reactions among combat soldiers in the 1982 Lebanon War. Much of that can be attributed to the vital instrumental role of the commanding officer in combat: he is the one who has the maps and plans, who knows what to do, and who gives the orders. To a great extent, the combat soldier's life depends on the competence of his commanding officer.

In the Gulf War, where soldiers saw no combat and their commanding officers knew little if anything more about the situation than they did and could do nothing to affect it, other elements of officer support apparently came into play in reducing stress. It seems that even on "the home front," the commander still served as a parent figure who could provide a role model and radiate a sense of authority, security, and control even where the objective situation was very uncertain. The finding in the navy study that distress was lower in units where the commanders held regular news briefings is interesting in this connection. The briefings for the most part were based on the same newspaper articles that every soldier could read for himself or herself. What evidently made the difference is not simply the information provided, but the order, structure, and care that the commanders gathering their soldiers together for joint discussion conveyed and, in part, created.

## Patients and Nonpatients

Both patients and nonpatients showed symptoms of stress. However, they differed in the severity of their symptomatology, their sense of self-efficacy, and their perception of social support, especially from their commanders.

First, patients showed higher levels of both general psychiatric and stress-related symptomatology than nonpatients. As noted above, considerably more patients than nonpatients reached outpatient levels on the SCL-90-R. In addition, with the exception of increased sensitivity to noise endorsed by about three-quarters of both groups, and hypervigilance, endorsed by over half of the nonpatients, a substantially smaller proportion of the nonpatients than patients endorsed the specifically stress-related symptoms in the 20-item checklist. Each of these symptoms (with the exception of somatic complaints) was endorsed by about half the patients but a much smaller proportion of the nonpatients. For example, 57% of patients reported recurrent thoughts about the war, in contrast to 40% of nonpatients; sleep problems, 57% versus 31%; difficulties in memory and concentration, 56% versus 22%; feeling distant from others, 45% versus 19%; feelings of panic, 45% versus 18%; and somatic complaints, 36% versus 13%. What we see here in the endorsement of individual symptoms is the same pattern of stress indicated by the average of the endorsements, with the patient group showing a moderate level and the nonpatient group a low level.

This finding is consistent with findings of prior studies both within and outside the military. Solomon (1989b), for example, found that posttraumatic combat veterans who sought psychiatric help had more severe psychiatric and somatic symptomatology and more problems in social functioning than posttraumatic veterans who did not. In civilian life, Nadler (1983) found that the severity of symptoms and how much they interfere with day-to-day functioning are among the decisive factors in people's seeking professional help. An explanation is suggested by Brickman, Rabinowitz, Karuza, Coates, Cohen, & Kidder's (1982) view that the first step in seeking help is the identification of a disturbance. Likely as not, soldiers' low-grade symptoms escaped the necessary identification and labeling, especially if they interfered only minimally with the soldiers' daily functioning.

Along with this, high levels of distress alone did not always result in help seeking. The sense of self-efficacy and social support that mitigated the level of distress soldiers reported also made them less inclined to ask for professional assistance. The nonpatients in the study not only had less severe symptomatology than the patients, but they also felt more able to cope on their own and reported more sources of social support. The support of commanding officers was particularly lacking among the patients. Asked to rank 11 potential sources of support in terms of how helpful they actually were during the war, nonpatients ranked their commanding officers in 5th place, while patients put them way down at the bottom of the list, in 11th place! These findings are also consistent with previous studies, which have shown that people's appraisal of their ability to cope with their problems on their own and their perception of whether alternative sources of help (such as friends, family, teachers, clergyman) are available and potentially effective both influence the decision to seek therapeutic assistance.

The patients also differed from the nonpatients in the higher proportion of reservists among them. Reservists in Israel are somewhat older soldiers, for the most part males, who have already completed their regular army service. Ranging in age from their early twenties to mid-fifties, many have families, jobs, businesses, and other activities and responsibilities that they leave behind when they go to reserve duty. While getting up and going to the army is a matter of routine for regular and career soldiers, for reservists it means a change, often quite disruptive, in their normal routine. This change can be stressful under any circumstances. Among other things, it may mean finding people to fill in for one at home and at work. It is likely to be all the more disruptive in wartime, when many men are in the army at the same time and replacements are hard to find. Earlier research in Israel has found that reservists also tend to be more susceptible than the younger regulars to combat stress reaction on the battlefield.

Conspicuous by their absence in the patient group were officers. There was not a single officer among the patients and, as noted above, not one of them even acknowledged feeling a need for treatment. This is consistent with prior findings of very low rates of acute combat stress reactions among officers during the 1982 Lebanon War (Solomon, Noy, & Bar-On, 1986). Officers are, of course, a select group. They all pass strict screening procedures that include evaluation not only of their intellectual and physical powers but also of their psychological health and resilience to stress. Moreover, both the special training they receive and their responsibilities may enhance their resistance to stress. The findings indicate that as a group they reported lower levels of distress than nonofficers. Moreover, officers also have good reason to cope by themselves with whatever distress they do feel. In their high positions, they have considerably more to lose than the ordinary soldier if they seek psychiatric help: namely, the respect of the soldiers under them, the esteem of their peers and others in their social milieu, and their own sense of who they are and what they can do. For all the changes of the posttherapeutic era, seeking psychological help still carries a stigma, especially in the army. For an officer to seek help for tensions of the Gulf War would be to confess weakness in precisely the area for which he or she was chosen and primed to perform. The price to be paid for doing that might outweigh the benefits.

Of those who applied to the IDF central mental health clinic during the war, only 60% reported that they needed psychological assistance. This apparent anomaly may be explained partly by denial and partly by the use of the mental health facilities for ulterior purposes. Prior studies have demonstrated that people do sometimes turn to medical and mental health services for reasons that fall outside the caregiving agency's official mandate. For instance, Israeli immigrants have been found to turn to medical services for companionship under the guise of needing treatment for a minor ailment (Shuval, Markus, & Dotan, 1973). In the army, mental health agencies may be misused to provide exit tickets for soldiers who want a legitimate out and cannot get it in any other way.

Unofficial clinical impressions were that many of the wartime "patients" at the mental health clinic were, in fact, seeking a temporary release from reserve duty, primarily out of concern for their families. They denied any personal distress and mostly applied to the mental health clinic after having failed to attain the cooperation of their commanding officers.

## A Job for Commanding Officers

Although it is obvious that commanding officers cannot be too free with the leaves they grant, especially in emergency situations, it remains that at least some of the problems presented to the IDF mental health clinic may more properly have been resolved by a compassionate commander willing to listen and assist with personal problems. Indeed, the findings of the study, as well as of the air force and navy investigations, suggest that commanding officers could have played a more positive role in reducing soldiers' distress during the Gulf War. They could have made much more of their position of authority to imbue their units with the sense of order and purpose that do so much to mitigate stress and to help people cope with danger and uncertainty. They could also have used their own behavior to provide a model of confidence and calm functioning for their soldiers and to encourage their active coping.

## HIGH MARKS IN TROUBLED TIMES

The three studies presented above were each conducted independently on different samples, in different branches of the IDF. Yet they present a consistent picture indicating that, on the whole, Israel's soldiers coped well during the Gulf War. In a situation where external problem-focused coping could provide little relief, they were apparently able to cope adaptively in other ways: by finding strength in their affiliation with the army and the nation, by turning to one another for social support, and by drawing on their own resources, namely their sense of perceived self-efficacy, to handle the crisis and their ability to control or externalize their stress through activity. They were thus able to cope not only with the risk of missile attack that they shared with ordinary citizens but also with numerous difficulties attendant on their being soldiers: the military's forced passivity, the sense of dissonance inherent in this departure from the traditional and expected IDF (and their own) response to threat, their worry about their families huddled in sealed rooms, and the confusion of instructions, especially at the war's start.

These findings were not altogether expected. Subjects in all three studies were sampled exclusively from bases in the center of the country—the area most often hit by the Scuds. Of all of Israel's soldiers, they were exposed to the greatest objective risk during the Gulf War. At the same time, they were probably the least fit to cope with that risk. Assignment to bases in the center of the country is generally restricted to soldiers with relatively low military fitness profiles who do not meet the criteria for admittance to the demanding combat units situated in the country's farther reaches.

Under the circumstances, it is not surprising that a small minority of soldiers experienced high levels of distress during the war and that some of them applied to IDF mental health clinics. These soldiers are the focus of the next two studies.

## STUDY 4: APPLICANTS TO THE CENTRAL IDF MENTAL HEALTH CLINIC

During the Gulf War, the IDF Central Mental Health Clinic remained open around the clock. This clinic provides all types of mental health services, except hospitalization, for regular, reserve, and career soldiers assigned to bases in Israel's central region. Since this was the most vulnerable part of the country during the Gulf War, the IDF's mental health research branch undertook to examine any possible changes in the rates and types of referrals to the clinic.

The study, conducted by Kaplan, Kron, Lichtenberg, Solomon, and Bleich (1992), revealed, first of all, that there was only a small increase in referrals: approximately 10% above normal.

The authors distinguished four main groups of clinic applicants whose problems related to the war: reserve soldiers who had compromised functioning before the war; regular soldiers with special service conditions due to emotional family problems; regular reserve soldiers with family problems; and soldiers with PTSD. Each of these groups is described briefly below.

### Reserve Soldiers with Compromised Functioning before the War

This group consisted mostly of reserve soldiers who had relatively easy and risk-free assignments in the Civil Defense Force or had been posted as guards in rear units because of some previous difficulty in military functioning, psychological or physical disability, family problems, or age. In previous wars, the risks were borne by younger and fitter soldiers fighting at the front, while soldiers such as these remained far from danger, patrolling the streets, maintaining public order, and enforcing blackouts. In this war, however, they suddenly found themselves in the areas most at risk for attack and unexpectedly called upon to perform tasks for which they were unprepared. They were often assigned to small teams with people they did not know and without a clear and available command structure in the field. Some were required to act as sentries on the roofs of tall buildings to scout areas where missiles might land; others had to go out to the landing sites when the missiles struck. These were potentially dangerous tasks that could make the soldiers close witnesses of destruction and exposed them to personal injury. These were dangers to which these soldiers had not been exposed in previous wars and which many of them were emotionally unprepared to handle in the Gulf War.

Their most frequent clinical complaints included acute anxiety, depression, despair, regressive behavior such as crying and hair pulling, and threats of suicide if they were not released from reserve duty. Some of these soldiers would curl up in the clinic waiting room and would not respond when their name was called. Others refused to wait their turn, demanding to be seen immediately.

## Regular Soldiers with Lenient Service Conditions

The second group consisted of younger soldiers doing their compulsory military service. Like the older applicants in the first group, these soldiers had also been deemed unsuitable for service at the front. Most of them were posted to rear guard units in the central region because of psychiatric, physical, or family problems. These soldiers also experienced acute distress when they were required to carry out more tasks, to function on a higher level, and to spend more time at their bases. Many of them had been accustomed to receiving a variety of unofficial privileges, such as home leaves, fewer hours on duty, and longer vacations, but their commanders could no longer bend the rules for them. Many of these regular soldiers who applied for help had character and adjustment problems. When they were confronted with increased demands and separated from their families and deprived of family support, they became depressed and anxious.

In treatment, these soldiers were presented with clear demands to adapt. They were informed that failure to comply would not bring them lighter duties but could lead to their discharge from the army, with all its social and occupational consequences in Israel. In some cases, their parents were called in to provide the treatment staff with information or to provide support for the soldier's proper functioning. Once the war was over, most of the soldiers in this category were able to fulfill their duties much better.

## Soldiers with Family Problems

The third group of patients included both regular and reserve soldiers who applied because of concern for their families. Most showed no serious psychopathology and had never before been treated in a mental health setting. This group was generally of a higher socioeconomic level than the previous two groups. Their typical complaint was an inability to carry out assignments because of concern about loved ones who were ill or otherwise unable to cope on their own. Frequently cited were wives and children who panicked with every alarm and dependent elderly parents. These soldiers believed that their families would not be able to manage without them. They rejected the idea that they themselves might have a problem, and did not request a release from service or a reduction in their military fitness rating. They insisted that they were healthy and that only their families' suffering was preventing them from properly carrying out their military duties. Generally, they applied to the mental health clinic only after their commanders and military welfare services were unable to help. Often they were able to return to full military functioning after a short leave.

## Traumatized Soldiers

The fourth group consisted of traumatized soldiers. In some cases, the trauma was induced by an incident in the Gulf War. More often, the traumatic event was in a previous war, terrorist incident, or training mishap, and the Gulf War simply triggered a reactivation of the prior stress. Some of the soldiers in this group had been successfully treated in the past for combat stress reaction; others had broken down and never returned to normal functioning, and their condition deteriorated further in the course of the war. Some of the soldiers in this category had to be discharged from the army.

In this war-torn country, many soldiers bear the scars of prior conflicts. For trauma victims, every new war brings repressed images and memories to the surface and aggravates ongoing distress. Even if such soldiers are not actively serving at the time, television news coverage of wartime events can be enough to trigger a reactivation. A poignant example of this involving a former Israeli pilot, Gideon Dror, whose plane had been shot down during the Six Day War in 1967, was reported in the Israeli press. When pictures of American and British prisoners of war (POWs) captured by the Iraqis were broadcast on television, Dror, who had been a POW in Iraq, told an Israeli newspaper of his deep sense of identification with the young pilots staring out at him from the television screen. He was especially distressed by seeing a pilot who abandoned his plane in the same spot where he himself had abandoned his 23 years earlier. The newscast reawakened in him the strong feelings of helplessness he experienced when he was captured and taken prisoner.

The soldiers who applied to the mental health clinic with PTSD symptoms during the Gulf War were the subject of the fifth study.

## STUDY 5: PTSD AMONG SOLDIERS DURING THE GULF WAR

During the Gulf War, 74 soldiers applied or were referred to the Unit for Treatment of Combat Stress Reactions in the Central Mental Health Clinic. They were studied by Kaplan, Singer, Lichtenberg, Solomon, and Bleich (1992), who attempted to group these patients in terms of the background and manifestations of their symptoms. The researchers found that of the 74 soldiers applying with PTSD symptoms, 72 had already had stress reactions to prior military events and that these were reactivated with the Gulf War. They distinguished four distinct groups of traumatized soldiers.

The largest group (30 soldiers, 40%) suffered from *severe generalized chronic sensitivity*. Even prior to the Gulf War, these soldiers had responded with stress to stimuli that, to all appearances, were unconnected with the original traumatogenic event. Such diverse and general stimuli as gatherings of people at parties or on the street, the sound of children at play, and the movement of traffic could provoke distress. That being the case, few if any areas of their lives were unaffected, and they suffered from ongoing PTSD symptoms. Moreover, some had developed phobic responses; some medicated themselves with alcohol or drugs; and some were under long-term pharmacotherapy. Disturbing enough in civilian life, in reserve duty, their symptoms often attained an intensity that completely inhibited their functioning. Six of them had been permanently released from reserve duty.

With the outbreak of the Gulf War, the men in this group complained of sleep difficulties, nightmares, anxiety, agitation, and uncontrollable outbursts of rage. Some reached the mental health clinic directly from their homes without being drafted. Others, who were drafted for service in the rear under the misapprehension that it was not as dangerous or anxiety provoking as service on the front, applied soon afterward. Eighteen of them were discharged during the war. Their release dramatically relieved their distress.

*Specific sensitivity* was displayed by 27 soldiers (37%). These men had low-intensity residual symptoms of prior PTSD, but in contrast to those who displayed generalized sensitivity, they were able to function well in most areas of civilian life. Moreover, although they had developed selective sensitivity to stimuli reminiscent of the original traumatic event, they also functioned competently in their peacetime reserve duty, many of them investing considerable effort to do so. As the Gulf War approached, however, their sensitivity to military stimuli intensified, and on receiving their call-up notices, most of them responded with strong anticipatory anxiety. When they reported for reserve duty, their previously mild symptoms were exacerbated, and they soon applied for mental health assistance.

Soldiers with *uncomplicated reactivation* (15, 20%) seemed to have recovered completely from their past stress reaction. They had no residual symptoms, and up to the Gulf War functioned well in both civilian life and reserve duty. Their reexposure to war, however, evidently unmasked a latent vulnerability and induced a stress reaction. Some of the men were afraid to report to their units, even to procure a referral to the clinic. Once in service, they became intensely anxious and depressed, lost their appetites, and were unable to sleep. They showed hypersensitivity to noise, were bothered by intrusive thoughts and memories of their previous traumatic experiences, and both their civilian and military functioning deteriorated. They expressed an implacable sense that their lives were in imminent danger, that no place was safe, and that they could do nothing to escape the threat. Most of these patients required intensive psychotherapy, and some received medication as well.

Only two of the patients (3%) who showed intensive stress reactions during the Gulf War had no known history of prior combat stress reaction or PTSD. As far as could be told, their reactions stemmed from the Gulf War alone.

The literature on posttrauma contains two opposing views of the type of stressor most likely to trigger reactivation. One holds that vulnerability to stress following PTSD is nonspecific, so that any stressor, however little it resembles the original one, may induce a reactivation. The other holds that the more similar the stressors, the greater the likelihood of reactivation. The categories that were found support both these views. Somewhat fewer than half the soldiers showed severe stress symptoms in response to a large range of stimuli even before the war; somewhat more than half developed severe symptoms with the onset of the war, which, by virtue of its being a specifically military stressor, more closely resembled the military situations in which they had first been traumatized.

## HELP-SEEKING FINDINGS

Two major findings emerge from the study of help seeking in the Gulf War. First, the IDF mental health facilities were not inundated with applicants; only 10% more than the unusual peacetime number applied for assistance. Second, with two notable exceptions, namely those who turned to the mental health facilities to obtain leave to take care of their families and the two soldiers who developed severe traumatic stress reactions without any known psychiatric breakdown in the past, treatment was sought mainly by soldiers with prior vulnerability. Almost all of those who developed severe stress reactions (Study 5) had prior breakdowns in combat, terrorist incidents, or training, and their responses in the Gulf War were clear cases of reactivation. Of the others, a good portion had either showed compromised functioning before the war or had personal problems that warranted lenient terms of service (Study 4).

It can be suggested that, by and large, the failure of these soldiers to function well in the past either continued into the Gulf War or depleted the energy, self-confidence, motivation, and other inner resources that might have helped them cope better with the challenges they faced. This suggestion is in keeping with the finding in Study 4 that help seeking was correlated with low perceived self-efficacy. It is also in keeping with Bandura's view that success fosters the sense of mastery that makes for further success, while failure leads to further failure by undermining the sense of mastery needed to motivate the person to invest the effort to succeed in a task (Bandura, 1977).

The findings are both similar to and different from those on help seeking among combat soldiers. The similarity is in the soldiers with reactivated traumas. Studies of combat soldiers in Israel also showed that soldiers with prior traumatic stress reactions were more likely to break down in a subsequent war than either novice soldiers or soldiers who had weathered earlier wars without psychiatric incident (Solomon, 1993). The difference has to do with possible predispositional factors. While studies of combat breakdowns have not found any predispositional factors that could predict which soldiers would break down and which ones would not (Solomon, 1993), Study 4 hints that soldiers with prior emotional problems were at risk. The difference may be that combat is traumatogenic by its very nature, while the Gulf War was merely stressful.

Nonetheless, one of the questions raised by these studies is why more soldiers did not seek help. Why was there only a 10% rise over peactime applications among a population of soldiers faced with stresses for which they had no prior preparation, either practical or emotional? The low incidence (4%) of "outpatient level" distress found among the nonpatient groups in Study 3 suggests that most of the soldiers who needed help may already have been receiving it when the Gulf War broke out. There is also the possibility that since the mental health clinic is located in the central region of the country, applying for help there would not have served to remove the soldiers from the high-risk area that provoked their anxiety, which is one of the functions of help seeking in combat (Solomon, 1993). On the other hand, it is also possible that the stigma attached to help seeking in the army may have deterred at least some of those who could have benefited from professional assistance. However, looked at yet another way, the very modest increase in help seeking, especially if the applicants who had ulterior motives are discounted, suggests that the IDF struck a successful balance of legitimizing help seeking and encouraging functioning.

# 10

# Mental Health Professionals in the Public Arena

The Gulf War saw a sudden surge in the public exposure of mental health professionals. The print and electronic media alike were inundated with psychiatrics, psychologists, and social workers offering information, advice, and just plain opinions having to do with the many emotional issues raised by the war. Others staffed well-publicized telephone hotlines established to answer callers' questions, calm their fears, and offer suggestions for handling the difficulties and dilemmas they encountered. Even as this was going on, though, there was a barrage of criticism from both laypersons and professionals about the role these practitioners played and the message they relayed. In retrospect, it became apparent that not all the implications of their conduct had been thought out and that, basically, no one had really given much consideration to the question of what the role of the mental health profession should be in a national crisis. This chapter will attempt to deal with the issue by looking closely at the various endeavors of the mental health profession during the war, focusing on contributions they made or did not make to public coping and morale.

## MENTAL HEALTH PROFESSIONALS AT LOOSE ENDS

We begin by looking at the personal situation that Israel's mental health professionals found themselves in during the war. While it is presumptuous to speak for all the members of these professions, it may be suggested that a good portion of them were underemployed and at loose ends.

Along with so much else in Israel at the time, private therapy was generally suspended. The emergency routine, which tied people to their homes and limited most out-of-house activity to daylight hours, made it difficult for patients to reach their therapists, while the life threat of the war tended to make the patients' intrapsychic conflicts seem paltry to them and out of place by comparison. Therapists, for their part, were reluctant to go on with their private clinical work. Writing of his own feelings during the war, the noted psychiatrist Dr. Max Stern (1992) tells of the difficulties of seeing patients during the war. He asked, "How can we deal with their problems? Can we be attentive to the fine tuning of their emotions in the present situation? Will we be able to relate seriously to what they tell us? Will we be able to empathize? to understand? to respond emotionally? What must we do when the external reality is more pressing than the internal world?" It was difficult for therapists, troubled by their own fears, to listen to their patients when they had "one ear tuned to a possible siren" and were thinking, "Is everything alright at home?" (p. 54).

Private practice in the therapist's home was particularly problematic. In the event of an alarm the therapist would find himself or herself and his or her family in the sealed room—often the bedroom—along with the patient, in violation of the neutrality that is generally considered essential to the therapeutic work. "What will happen then?" Stern asked. "How will it affect the patient to be brought, most concretely, into our bedroom, the sanctum of sanctums? He or she will be there with our wife and kids, will see how everyone in the family reacts to the threat of the missiles, will uncover those deep secrets that therapists usually hide from patients. What will the patient think, imagine, fantasize?" (p. 54).

The upshot was that therapists were no more eager than most of their patients to meet. As Stern puts it, somewhat bluntly, "What we in fact wanted to say was stay home until it's all over. We have no interest in your problems or wish to treat you. . . . I want to be with myself and my family. You're bothering me, imposing on me. You're not wanted" (p. 54).

In previous wars, therapists had been drafted to the front, where they provided front-line treatment to soldiers with combat stress. Dangerous as their work in the battle zone was, Stern tells, they felt fortified in knowing that they had an important job to do and how to do it. In the Gulf War, his absorption in his own anxieties and his confessed disinclination to see his patients constituted a blow to his self-image as a therapist. "Essential questions about my identity, my identity as a thera-

pist, come up. Who am I?" he asked himself. "Am I really a therapist?
. . . How can I be so egocentric, thinking only of my own little world?
Where is my dedication? My commitment? My desire to help? . . . I feel
ashamed. . . . Everything that I've built up over so many years, with such
hard work, was crumbling, disintegrating. Where was my true self?"

   The discomfiture Stern describes was probably shared by many
therapists, since it grew out of the nature of the war rather than out of
any personal idiosyncrasies. How much this discomfiture contributed to
the eagerness of mental health professionals to mount the public stage
can only be conjectured. What is clear, though, is that many professionals suddenly found themselves with time to spare and under emotional
stress that could conceivably have sought an outlet in the kind of war-
related public activities that they undertook. At the same time, it would
be doing an injustice to discount the well-documented human urge to
help out in disasters. In fact, a not dissimilar spate of activity by mental
health professionals was recorded in the wake of the 1985 Mexico City
earthquake (Palacios, Cueli, Camacho, Cleriga, Cuevas, & Cossof, 1986)
when professionals spontaneously threw themselves into the psychological training of rescue workers, set up programs to help schoolchildren
cope with the catastrophe, counseled the public over radio and television, and so forth. It can be argued that in the Gulf War, the two motives
coalesced.

## FROM PRIVATE PRACTICE TO THE PUBLIC ARENA

   Mental health professionals were active during the war in numerous
public arenas. This chapter will look at a number of the activities, including those on telephone hotlines, in public institutions like schools and
the army, and, most prominently, in the print and electronic media. The
coverage is neither comprehensive nor necessarily representative, but
should give some idea of the diversity and dimensions of the public role
the mental health profession played in the war.

### Telephone Hotlines

   During the war, a large number of hotlines, most of them staffed by
volunteer mental health professionals, were set up to serve various segments of the public who were perceived as having special needs. There
were hotlines for new immigrants, for the aged, for Holocaust survivors,
for students, and so forth. They provided authoritative information and
advice for people who sought solutions to immediate, war-related prob-

lems and who did not have easy access to information or help elsewhere. For example, the hotlines for the country's recent Russian arrivals provided much-needed guidance in their native language. Another hotline was set up by Nitzan, an organization for children with learning disabilities, when its offices were closed because of the emergency routine. Other hotlines were similarly set up on an impromptu basis to fill in for services that were curtailed in the war.

One of the largest, best-planned hotlines was that established by the Ministry of Education. This was a children's hotline, set up in September, four months prior to the outbreak of the war, by Dr. Bilha Noy, director of the Ministry of Education Open Line for Students (Noy B., 1991), and went into operation with the closure of the schools on the morning of January 16, 1991. The idea behind the hotline was that with the schools closed, children were deprived of their natural source of support and leadership just when they most needed it. The hotline was established to fill the gap and to maintain the connection with the child's former anchor. It served as a source of information couched in terms children could understand, an outlet for the children's anxieties, and a source of advice, reassurance, and assistance in cases where the child's parents may not have been coping adequately with the situation.

Judging from the information provided in the report written by Dr. Bilha Noy, the hotline apparently strove to strike a balance between legitimizing students' expressions of fear and anxiety, on the one hand, and providing the kind of information, advice, and support that would bolster their coping and control, on the other.

This can be seen, for example, in the responses to the many expressions of anxiety that the hotline received. An elementary school child who called in to say, "Every time I hear an alert my body begins to shake, and I'm very embarrassed about it, but can't stop it," was reassured with the following explanation: "Most people feel tense and frightened when the alert sounds. Different people express this fear in different ways: some shake, others have diarrhea, another feels his heart thumping, and yet others feel nausea and even throw up. These are all normal reactions to a dangerous situation." At the same time, the child was told, "Your reaction shows that you are aware of the danger, and if you are aware of it you will also do something about it" (Noy B., 1991, p. 21).

According to the report, the hotline supported instrumental coping and discouraged regression and escape. The advice presented in the report seems to support this claim. Children who complained that they were afraid to go into the sealed rooms and wear their masks were given information about how to put on the mask and assured that they were safer in that room than anywhere else during an alert. When the schools reopened, children who were afraid to walk there or to go on their own were advised (depending on their age) to ask their parents to drive them or to organize a carpool with some of their friends. They were told, "Try to overcome your fear even if you'd rather be at home" (p. 26). Where children complained of parents who panicked or did not seal a room or wear their mask, the parents were spoken to and told, "Your child feels anxious when you do not follow instructions." Parents were reminded that their job was to keep their kids calm (Noy B., 1991, p. 21). Children who asked what to do if there was an alert on the way to school were advised, "Since you have your mask with you, the first thing to do is to put it on. If a missile lands in the area, fall to the ground. If not, walk slowly (the mask blurs your vision) to the nearest shelter" (Noy B., 1991, p. 23).

Noy notes that the hotline was quite popular. The first day of the war there were so many calls that three additional lines were added, and another four lines were added three days later. The number of calls varied with the circumstances and the amount of media exposure the service received. Some days hundreds of calls were received, others, thousands.

Unlike the other public activities of mental health professionals, their work on the hotlines was not called into question. As long as their exchanges and advice remained private and were not published or broadcast, the hotlines were seen as providing an important public service, as meeting the specific needs of the people who turned to them, and as not having much, if any, negative overflow.

## Mental Health Activities in Large Public Institutions

Mental health professionals were also active in institutions such as hospitals, schools, and the Israel Defense Forces (IDF). We have three presentations of work with large public institutions: one describing interventions in the Haifa school system, and two describing interventions in the IDF. These illustrate some of the activities that were undertaken, the problems they were meant to address, and the problems they themselves entailed.

The intervention in the Haifa school system is the most convincing of the three. Organized by Rina Meisels (unpublished manuscript), senior educational psychologist in the service department of the Haifa municipality and clinical psychologist at a Haifa general hospital, the intervention consisted of workshops for teachers and school staff. The design was based on Meichenbaum's (1985) notion of "stress inoculation and acquired immunity," which holds that people who are preacquainted

with the obnoxious characteristics of a stress situation are better able to
deal with it when it occurs. The workshops were started before the war
broke out, and there was a second round during the war after the
schools reopened.

As Meisels describes them, the workshops began with an airing of
the participants' fears; moved on to a more theoretical discussion of
stress and its cognitive, behavioral, emotional, and somatic manifestations in both children and adults; and from there proceeded to the main
issue for that audience: the schoolchildren. The participants worked on
how to talk to the children about the situation; how to deal with difficulties created by the gas masks (such as trouble breathing, reluctance to
put it on, the sense of impersonality and discipline problems it evoked);
and how to alleviate the children's tension by means of simple relaxation
techniques, humor, and creative and other activities, including volunteer work. The content of the workshops varied somewhat with grade
level, with regressive tendencies discussed in elementary schools and
abstract issues in high schools.

The workshops were supplemented with practical measures. In every school an "emergency team" consisting of the principal, the school
psychologist, the security guard, and the school nurse was established to
devise a plan for passing the time in the shelters should an alarm sound
during school time. Moreover, during the school closures, teachers were
instructed to telephone each of their pupils to see how they were. When
the schools were reopened more workshops were held, which addressed
the teachers' current anxieties and the problems that arose with the
falling Scuds, including those of people whose homes were hit.

Two projects were also launched by the IDF Mental Health Department. Ordinarily, mental health officers have their hands full in wartime
dealing with emergency mental health needs both on the front and in
the rear-echelon facilities where combat stress reaction casualties are
sent. In this war, where no shots were fired, these trained professionals
found themselves spending many hours at their bases without their usual client load and no alternative occupation. At the same time, some of
them felt that there was a great deal of tension around them, stemming
both from the direct threat of the war and from the soldiers' conflicting
responsibilities, discussed earlier, toward the army and their families.

One of the projects consisted of workshops set up after the first
Scud attack. The workshops were run by mental health teams. Most of
them were held in units in the center of the country, which were believed
to be at high risk for stress because of their location in the eye of the
storm and because the soldiers serving in them were deemed to be
somewhat problematic. The workshops generally consisted of a lecture

and discussion that presented the manifestations of anxiety, defined them as normal, and presented techniques for stress reduction and, later on for those who wanted them, relaxation exercises. The idea was that enabling soldiers to vent and work out any natural war-related stress in this way would reduce the need for formal referrals to the mental health clinics, with the resultant danger of stigmatization, and also would help commanders to identify and deal with their troops' stress symptoms.

According to Saul Guri, a veteran mental health social worker on staff at the Career Officers' Mental Health Clinic who was active in these workshops, the workshops conveyed a double message: "It's legitimate to be anxious, and you can cope with your anxiety" (Guri, 1992, January). Guri claims that the participants reacted positively. Though the traditionalists in the department felt that the active, unsolicited outreach overstepped the bounds proper to the profession and that clients should be the ones to approach professionals and not the other way around, Guri insists that there was a genuine need. "Some officers shut themselves up in their offices and hardly functioned. As soon as they knew about us they were very happy." On the other hand, only one commander actually asked for a workshop for his unit of his own initiative, and one workshop was canceled because only two officers showed up. The disparity may be explained by the fact that the project was organized ad hoc under the pressure of the missile strikes without any examination of the prevalence of the need.

A second project was launched by Lieutenant Colonel Chen Nardi, a mental health officer and social worker. Nardi wrote and distributed a small, pocket-sized guide to stress management. Called *The Tranquilizer,* the easy-to-use guide was based on cognitive–behavioral principles. Each page or two was devoted to a particular stress management technique, with examples and instructions for using it. The techniques listed were guided imagery (for example, "Imagine yourself in the midst of a pleasant experience. . . ."); self-talk (for example, "Say to yourself, 'I won't let my fear get the better of me, I'll control it'"); relaxation; and constructive activities such as talking with friends and helping others. The booklet was initially distributed to soldiers, usually at the end of stress-reduction workshops. Later, revised editions were distributed to commanders to help them handle the stress of their subordinates, as well as to groups in the civilian population.

The booklet came under a great deal of criticism, to say nothing of ridicule, both within and outside the army. Its simple messages made it easy to make fun of. Also, it assumed a level of stress that was never proved and addressed the readers at the low end of their maturity and intellect. The various covers of the booklet, one containing a drawing of a dragon, another of a peaceful house, and so forth, were absurdly childish and did nothing to enhance the maturity or courage of the people to whom they were addressed. Noy (Noy S., 1991) objected that the very aim of the booklet was misguided, since the war situation called for vigilance, not calm.

Nardi (1992, January) admits that the booklet was his "own personal way of coping" with the anxiety he felt, but defends it on the grounds that "when it was needed it worked." Whether or not that is the case, we are not in a position to say. However, in its defense, the booklet did catch on. Generals were seen carrying it like a talisman in their shirt pockets, and civilian institutions such as banks actually asked for editions for their employees.

## The Media

The most controversial area of mental health activity was the media. To be sure, the Gulf War is certainly not the first war in Israel in which the media played an important mental health role on the home front. In the 1973 Yom Kippur War, for example, the media met a range of public needs, among them emotional ones. According to Peled and Katz (1974), the media met public needs not only for information and interpretation of events, for reinforcement of national solidarity, and for participation in the mourning of the war dead, but also for social connectedness and relief from anxiety. Dotan and Cohen (1976) similarly found that in addition to meeting the usual needs for escape and the augmented wartime needs for information and interpretation and for reinforcement of trust in the nation's leaders and pride in the country and army, the media met *affective needs*, among them that of raising morale.

But the Gulf War was certainly the first war in which the media virtually handed over to psychologists, educators, and other professionals the task of meeting the public's wartime mental health needs. During the 1967 Six Day War, to take a contrasting example, the task of maintaining public morale was carried out by the then head of intelligence, Chaim Herzog. In the guise of "national information supplier," Herzog broadcast a daily report whose objective was to calm the public. During the Gulf War, the army spokesman Nachman Shai was popularly known as the "national tranquilizer," and his spectacled face and soothing voice were featured regularly on radio and television. But the psychologists stole the show.

In small measure, psychologists were brought into the media by the military. Following the first Scud alarm in the small hours of January 19, when nobody at the joint radio station knew what the siren meant or what to do, military psychologists were brought in along with some senior journalists to provide guidelines for wartime broadcasting.

Most of the initiative, however, came from the media itself. On the simplest level, there was the need to fill space when war news was limited and, to quote an editor of a leading morning newspaper, mental health issues made for "spicy" reading (Cohen, Brog, Cheffer, Paz, Raviv, & Witztum, 1992, p. 17). More seriously, according to a study by Akiba Cohen and colleagues (1992) on mental health and the mass media during the Gulf War, the broadcasters themselves felt that discussion of problems growing out of the war was in order, but they did not quite know how to go about it or what advice to give. So they called on experts to speak on talk shows and phone-ins. Similarly, print journalists actively sought out educators and psychologists to interview, while, from the other direction, there were mental health professionals who wrote articles and letters to the editor.

A good part of the motivation of both the media and the professionals who responded to the courtship stemmed from the nature of the war itself. With Israel not engaged militarily, the war on the home front was largely a war of nerves. After attending to the news (or what passed for news) of the front, to the monitored accounts of the missile damage in Israel, and to the exhaustive and exhausting analyses that were offered up on the political and military aspects of the war, people were left with their concrete problems—how to get recalcitrant children to put on their gas masks, how to pass the tense time in the sealed room, and how to cope with their tension and anxieties.

The usual government and military authorities were not in a position to address these issues. They were out of their depth, their extensive denial before the war made them suspect, and there really was no single public figure in Israel who had the confidence and respect of enough of the public to be effective. As far as the public was concerned, there was a marked lack of government leadership. The leadership style of the then prime minister, Yitzhak Shamir, was notably laconic and stone-faced, while his ministers had engaged in too much ugly public infighting to inspire confidence.

Mental health professionals were asked to fill the vacuum. As Stern (1992) observes rather sardonically, "The establishment gave us a stage. . . . The 'adults' in the government up there above don't know what to do. We hear pronouncements and counter-pronouncements. No one takes responsibility, no one is at the helm. . . . Instead they find people in our profession to speak to the nation. . . . Salvation is in our hands" (pg. 56). The editor of a major afternoon paper unabashedly admitted that "we are the couch on which the public can get its therapy" (Cohen et al., 1992, p. 13).

Mental health workers were already making media appearances on war-related matters during the long waiting period before the start of the fighting. When the missiles began to fall, they became media darlings. A welter of advice, explanations, and reassurances could be seen, heard, and read, especially in the war's early days. This represented a significant shift in the role that the mental health profession played in Israel. To be sure, the ground had been prepared much earlier. In the decade prior to the war, Israelis had become accustomed to mental health professionals, mainly psychologists, but also social workers, educators, and others, discussing family conflicts, male–female relationships, child rearing, education, sex, and so forth in print and on the airwaves. According to Klonoff (1983), they served not only as advice givers, but also as consumer educators and social commentators. Despite this, until the Gulf War, their presence in the media was relatively moderate. On radio they were heard mainly in the early morning and late night hours, presumably addressing pensioners, housewives, and night owls. In the print media, they were represented mainly in women's magazines and in magazines for the adolescent market. There were no equivalents of "Dear Abby" or "Dr. Ruth" in daily newspapers. Until the war, there was nothing like the flooding of the media with mental health issues that one finds regularly in the United States. With the war, however, mental health professionals were thrust into prominence, and they assumed, temporarily at least, a leadership role for part of the general population.

It is impossible to cover the entire content of their communications. Roughly, however, two interrelated types of communication can be discerned. One was normative. People were repeatedly informed that their anxiety was normal under the circumstances, that sleep problems and other somatic complaints were common responses to stress, that lots of children were afraid to put on their gas masks, that other people also had trouble breathing with the masks on, and so forth. The intent of such communication was to calm, to reassure, and to link people to others. The message was that their feelings and behavior were not pathological under the circumstances.

The second type, closely linked to the first and often found in the same communication, was up-front advice on practical problems raised by the war. The flavor of much of it can be illustrated by a newspaper interview with one of the Israeli leading psychiatrists, Dr. Samuel Tyanno, director of Geah Psychiatric Hospital and head of the Children's and Youth Department there (Namir, 1991). Asked whether a frightened child should be permitted to sleep with its parents, he suggested that there was no need to lose one's head because of the war and that it was a better idea for the parent to sit at the child's bedside and calm him or her down. Asked what to do about bedwetting, he pointed out that it was a normal reaction to stress even among older children, and suggested that the parent should simply change the child's pajamas and reassure him or her that it happens to others as well. His advice, like so much other advice that was given during this period, was largely pragmatic and to the point and was targeted to specific questions that evidently taxed enough of the public for them to be dealt with in a newspaper.

One of the major thrusts of the communication was to legitimize the anxiety that people were feeling when they did not know when or where the next missile would fall and whether it would carry a conventional or an unconventional payload. This was done directly and unabashedly. The following are only a few examples:

I think that it's quite legitimate that a child, in these strange circumstances, should cry. Let's imagine ourselves as adults in the sealed room. Maybe we don't cry, but often when a child does not have the verbal ability to ask or get a verbal explanation, he reacts by crying. Crying when there are familiar people around is helpful. (Radio broadcast, January 18, 1991; Dr. Raviv, psychologist, cited in Cohen et al., 1992)

Fear should be given legitimization because there is existential anxiety, and it cannot be ignored. The legitimization should be given to adults, for an anxious adult passes on the message to children. Telling children not to be afraid is inappropriate when parents convey their own fear. (Bina Weiler, rehabilitation psychologist, quoted in Knoller, 1991b)

Just about the most foolish thing that can be done now . . . is to fear anxiety. Anxiety during wartime is an adaptive response; that is, it is an entirely natural response that arises in a situation where there is a real life threat. If at all, I'd be worried about someone who wasn't anxious. People who aren't anxious make me wonder why they're so blocked. Are they denying, repressing, unable to deal with the situation? At the same time, the anxiety mustn't turn into . . . panic. Panic, loss of control, can cause the person, instead of taking responsibility for himself and his children and taking the right steps to defend his life, to do just the opposite. (Interview with Dr. Shabtai Noy, by Livni, 1991)

Feelings of anxiety and regressive reactions of the Israeli population are legitimate and are experienced by virtually everyone. Those who are not anxious are the exception. They usually suffer from megalomania, and may even be considered psychopathic and relentless criminals. Every person who reacts with stress and anxiety, and reacts in his own individual way, is motivated by love, worry or some similar feeling. (Lavie J., 1991)

Such assertions tread a thin line. For the most part their major message was that anxiety was not pathological under the circumstances. The statements were part, often a small part, of larger communications whose thrust tended to be practical and oriented toward instrumental coping. For example, in the same newspaper piece in which she tells that anxiety should not be denied and cautions against double messages, Bina Weiler (Knoller, 1991b) emphasizes the role of information, support, and activity in mitigating tension, and advises parents to deal with any psychosomatic manifestations of anxiety in their children by having their family doctor examine the children. Similarly, while the psychologist Shabtai Noy of the Hebrew University in Jerusalem declares that anxiety is reasonable under the circumstances, he warns against giving it such free rein that it turns into panic. He suggests that the message psychologists relay to the public be that "the second night [of missile attacks] is easier than the first because we are learning to adjust and getting experience." He also offers practical suggestions for dealing with the anxiety, such as installing a telephone in the sealed room and pairing up with someone else if you are living alone.

Some of the statements, however, crossed the line. Joshua Lavie, the author of the pointedly titled *In Praise of Anxiety* (1991), for example, was rather heavy-handed in calling everyone who did not feel anxiety a megalomaniac and near criminal. He also bent over backward to justify some of the less mature expressions of the fear. Warning that anxiety can become dysfunctional when it has insufficient outlets in action, as was the case during the Gulf War, he expatiates at some length:

> This is why it is important to give the Israeli public legitimization [for its anxiety] and even to encourage regulating anxiety during this period. The gradual return to an "emergency routine" is one such control. The intra-city wandering between friends and relatives and hotels is another. As long as these actions do not involve criminal acts, they should be accepted. As time goes by, people will become accustomed to the situation and their reactions will change.
>
> Anxiety is also expressed in regressive modes of behavior. . . . For example, a person who finds himself in unexpected danger will cry out "mommy" or "oh god"; he will tremble all over, as children do, and probably revert back to his mother tongue, even if he does not usually use it. This regression is not retreat for the sake of retreat. It is the organism preparing to face danger, its mobilization of physical and emotional resources from the past and present. If an individual was used to eating or smoking at times of stress, he will probably feel the urge to do so again. If he was in the habit of hiding, then he will hide. On the other hand, if he was accustomed to danger, he will probably be found on the roof watching the missiles fly by. It is much easier to accept regression in children and in the aging in the face of danger, but to accept it in ourselves, as adults, is very difficult. (Lavie J., 1991)

Here the author has gotten carried away by his theme. Even if regression sometimes does serve the function of reorganization and advance, one may question the wisdom of legitimizing rooftop ventures to watch falling Scuds or even the less obviously dangerous activities of overeating, crying "mommy," and city hopping. Most of the opinions expressed by the various psychologists and their colleagues in other branches of the mental health community were considerably more balanced and better thought out.

## TAKE A GIANT STEP BACK: THE CRITICISM

There was extensive criticism of the role the mental health professionals played during the war. The criticism, which started during the war itself and snowballed afterward, came both from journalists and from mental health professionals, in many cases from professionals who themselves had jumped on the media bandwagon. As Stern (1992) describes it, there was a kind of embarrassment as the professionals realized that they had overextended themselves and were operating out of their own fears: "Slowly we climb off the stage, a bit embarrassed, asking pardon. We did what we were asked to do, we did our best, but. . . . We are undergoing a process of deflation. We're retreating and trying to say that essentially we're no different from anyone else. We're also afraid, we're also anxious, we're also helpless" (Stern, 1992, p. 56).

The basic objection was that the mental health professionals who ventured into the public realm somehow legitimized, spread, augmented, or even created the public's anxiety. Exactly what they were supposed to have done, and how, varied from critic to critic, but the overall and very widespread feeling was that they somehow contributed to the atmosphere of fear that pervaded the country during the war. At the least, they were accused of legitimizing fear, either by what they said or by the mere fact of their giving so much attention to the emotion. The point was repeatedly made that the constant preoccupation with and references to fear, stress, trauma, anxiety and anxiety symptoms, problems in the sealed room, and so forth in daily newspapers and over television and radio gave problems in coping and negative emotions undesirable emphasis and legitimacy. More harshly, mental health professionals were accused of creating a self-fulfilling prophecy, either on their own or as pawns of the media, by first broadcasting predictions that people would feel anxiety and the expected symptoms and then by advising them on measures to counter their tension. The general feeling can be summed up in the words of Professor Kalman Benyamini, a senior Israeli psychologist with an impressive record in public service: "Too many psychologists said too many things in too many places during this war that wasn't even a war for us" (Katzman, 1991).

Roughly, the criticism had two broad thrusts. One was against *what* the professionals did and did not say. The other was broader and ranged

over various issues involved in their public role, including the applica-
tion of the clinical approach to the general public, the inevitable distortions of the media, and the knotty question of whether mental health
professionals should have mounted the public stage at all. Below, I present and discuss the major objections.

## THE CONTENT: SINS OF COMMISSION AND OMISSION

### Overemphasis on Expression of Fear

One of the major criticisms of the content of the messages was that
they overemphasized the value of expression as a means of coping with
fear. One contention was that encouraging people to express their fear
could lead to panic if no one was around to calm them down. Professor
David Navon, winner of the Israel Prize for Psychology, made this a
central point of the report on coping with disasters, which he wrote for
the IDF after the war. In an appendix entitled "Public Fear Legitimization" (1992), he observed that while "expressing fears may help to avoid
symptoms that otherwise would be developed if the stress was repressed
or denied, . . . when the process is not supervised by a professional, and
professional aid is not readily available, ventilation may get out of control and turn into an overflow of anxiety, with possible chain reactions"
(pp. 180–183). Similar arguments were put forth against the advice that
parents encourage their children to cry or voice their fears (Katzman,
1991).

More comprehensively, Dr. Shabbtai Noy argued in his book *I Can
Not Anymore* (1991) that the expression of emotion is neither the only way
to cope with stress nor a desirable way when there is a real external
threat, as there was during the Gulf War. As he put it, when the house is
on fire, it is more important to bring water than to discuss one's feelings.
In support of this view he referred to information accumulated in military psychiatry and research in the field of civilian reactions to disasters.

### Neglect of Other Coping Methods

A corollary of the criticism of the professionals' emphasis on emotional expression is the claim that they neglected other means of coping.
Both Shabbtai Noy (1991) and Navon (1992) argued that it was erro-
neous to rule out denial. Noy, apparently forgetting the view he expressed in the newspaper interview he gave at the beginning of the war
that people who denied their fear were not able to cope (see above,
p. 20), suggested that as long as it did not interfere with functioning,

denial was as good as any other means of managing fear. Navon expressed concern that because of the public legitimization of fear, "People who did not experience or manifest fear might feel that they are abnormal" (p. 181).

Extending these arguments, Dr. Arik Shalev (1991b) and Dr. Eitan Bachar (1991) held that the communications on the media did not do justice to how varied the human response to stress is and that totally different responses, including mechanisms like partial denial, repression, and isolation, which are considered counterproductive and signs of problems in the clinical setting, may be functional for different people under different circumtances.

## No Message of Courage and Active Coping

A related and perhaps more fundamental criticism is that in times of crisis the task of the professional is to encourage courage and active coping. Article after article expresses the view that in responding to the public's fears, the professionals gave short shrift to the other half of the picture: the public's ability and need to cope. For example, the journalist Shulamit Har-Even (1991) objected that "there is too much talk here about hysteria and panic as an inevitable response and not enough about the other alternatives." The psychologist Dr. Dan Rudi (1991), who had participated in a radio phone-in during the war, made the point that for the general public, encouragement of courage and modes of overcoming fears would have been preferable to legitimizing anxiety.

Similarly Shabtai Noy (1991) contended that there was too much emphasis on calming the public's fears and not enough on active coping. As he sees it, the mental health professional's job in a threatening situation like the Gulf War is not to keep people calm, but rather to encourage them to stay alert, to trust in the national leadership, to follow the emergency regulations, to keep abreast of information, and to use active means of coping not only with their anxieties but with the external threat.

## BROADER ISSUES

### Help for the Few Harms the Many

With respect to the broader issues, one of the major criticisms was that the advice of the professionals was directed to only a very small minority of the population who had serious problems managing their anxiety. Most of the public, it was argued, could handle the tensions engendered by the war on their own, and those who could not should have been referred to therapy (Rudi, 1991). Navon (1992), in his careful analysis of the advantages and disadvantages of the mental health profession's legitimization of fear during wartime, insisted such legitimization has value, if at all, only for high-risk segments of the population. For most of the population, he contended, public legitimization was decidedly counterproductive. Speaking theoretically, he suggested that it could trigger or exacerbate people's anxiety by creating the expectation that they would not be able to cope with the stress on their own. The result, he warned, could be less effective coping and the generalization of anxiety, especially in borderline populations who would otherwise have controlled their fears.

In concrete terms, this line of criticism means that all the articles, talk shows, and phone-ins that dealt with specific problems and answered specific questions did more harm than good and should not have been offered at all. For every person who may have been helped by any given piece of advice, many more were harmed by the power of suggestion inherent in its publication. Basic to this objection is the idea that messages that are appropriate when addressed to patients in the privacy of the therapeutic setting are inappropriate and even damaging to the normal, nonpathological population reached through the media.

## The Media

All of the above criticisms are inextricably tied up with the well-known problems of what happens to messages when they are transmitted via the popular media.

In this connection, it is worth pointing out that none of those who criticized the health professionals' messages actually analyzed the contents of their statements. As was noted above, much, perhaps even most, of the advice was common sense and encouraged sensible, instrumental solutions to problems that came up. What the criticisms refer to are the *perceptions* of what was written and said, not to the actual contents. No one actually looked, for example, at how often expression of anxiety was encouraged and how often constructive ways of channeling or dealing with the emotion were counseled. The bulk of the criticism focused on the general sense of what came across. This sense did not necessarily reflect the professionals' intentions or statements. But any possible distortion is beside the point. What matters is that, accurate or not, the perceptions were widely held, both inside and outside the profession.

This is where the media comes in. Whatever was actually written or said, the nature of the media contributed to distorting the message and emphasizing any dysfunctional aspects it may have had. This can be readily seen in the newspaper headlines, which tended to draw attention to only the most simplistic and sensational aspects of advice that was generally much more subtle and balanced. For example, the level-headed advice in the Professor Samuel Dr. Tyanno interview (discussed above) was carried under the sensationalizing title "To Wake a Scream-ing Child from a Nightmare?" and the interview in which Shabtai Noy took pains to offer suggestions for active coping was headlined "Don't Be Afraid of Fear."

A deeper problem, hinted at above and noted by many of the critics, was that the very fact of discussing problems of anxiety in the media carried the danger of spreading it. As an example, we can take the article entitled "Helping Your Kids Get Back on Track" (Katzanelson, 1991, p. 7), in which the clinical and educational psychologist Edna Katzanelson advises parents on how to deal with various anxiety symp-toms that "might appear even after the danger passes." Her advice in-cludes such instrumental and commonsense guidelines as to create a calm atmosphere and avoid conflicts before bedtime to help children who might have problems sleeping; to help children who are exhibiting regressive behavior to resume age-appropriate conduct; and to commu-nicate to children who are suffering from psychosomatic pains that they have it within their power to overcome them. In relaying this advice, however, the author inevitably lists and predicts symptoms, and so pro-vides a basis for undesirable modeling.

It is essentially the media's enormous power of suggestion that made the critics recoil from the "public therapy" provided during the Gulf War. The clinical psychologist Dan Rudi, who manned a radio phone-in during the war, focused his critique of the professional's role on the issue of what happens when the private business of therapy goes public. His major criticism was that the phone-in he manned, by its very nature, spread fear. In his view, the open line served the minority of the population who could not manage their fear on their own, and that in providing them with a public forum in which to discuss their fear, the line made their problem public—and contagious. The same could obvi-ously be said of the advice offered in newspapers. This concern led him to urge, unsuccessfully, that the phone-in be suspended.

Like Rudi, Benyamini (cited in Katzman, 1991) is also concerned with the inevitable media distortion of the message conveyed by psychol-ogists. In his view, the psychologists who appeared in the media were not sensitive to how they came across or to the interpretation to which their assertions lent themselves. Benyamini does not go into detail, but he argues feelingly and forcefully that in appearing on the media, psychologists overstepped the bounds of the profession, misused their authority, and conveyed the message that people could not cope with their difficulties on their own:

> When a psychologist says something, there is added weight, added meaning to the words. . . . It doesn't matter how banal what you say is, it is accepted as the words of a man of science and not simply common sense. So [the message here is that] you can't do this on your own. You can't simply use your own intuition, common sense, family practices, or prayer. You need a professional for this. Using professionals [in the media] creates a paradoxical situation, where the message conveyed to the public is that "this is our business"—a message of dysfunction and incompetence. (Katzman, 1991, p. 16)

## A Time for Moralists, Not Psychologists

Of all the objections, the most far-reaching was that the Gulf War was a time for moralists, not psychologists. Behind this criticism is the feeling that the psychological approach, with its focus on pathology, its emphasis on personal as opposed to societal well-being, and its professed neutrality of values, is inappropriate, even damaging, in times of national crisis. There were recurrent objections to the applications of specific therapeutic techniques (especially free expression) to the general public, but the fundamental criticism cut much deeper.

It is expressed quite clearly by the journalist Sever Plotzker (1991). Plotzker criticizes the legitimization of fear at the expense of values and social cohesion. He regards the developments during the war as dangerous to a country of Israel's size and security situation, and attributes them to what he sees as the egotism and lack of commitment to values inherent in the psychological approach. Writing about two and a half weeks into the war, he argued that what was called for was moral leadership, not psychological counseling:

> I'm troubled by the fact that fear of the missiles has become a norm, a model for behavior. In this war, it's nice to be afraid. If being afraid is acceptable, then so are panic, hoarding, indifference to others. By this proud surrender to fear, we broadcast to ourselves and our friends egotism, helplessness, frustration and, above all, a lack of values. And not only a lack of national values but also a lack of social cohesion. A month ago I was sure that if a missile hit my home I would be able to count on my neighbors for help; today I'm not so certain. After all, we've all been given permission to act according to the dictates of our fear: that is, after the missile falls, to look out for our own skins only. . . .
> . . . It seems to me that in this war we have too many psychologists and too few philosophers, men of morals. We need someone to stand up and explain that if fearful behavior becomes routine in time of emergency, we will lose our homeland in Israel.

Very similar objections are raised from within the profession by

Kalman Benyamini (Katzman, 1991). Benyamini voices many of the reservations listed above. Among other things, he objects to the focus on expression as a means of moderating stress and is wary of the implications of giving psychological advice through the media. At bottom, however, his objections are much more comprehensive. He is concerned not only about the role that mental health professionals played in the war but about what he regards as the psychologization of the culture that was behind the profession going public. In his view, the "new culture," which promotes talking about personal problems and seeking psychological assistance for them, "entails a decline in social and political commitment. Everyone for himself and his personal search." He observes that his generation, which survived a succession of wars in which the existential danger was actualized, kept their fears to themselves, if they had any, and relied on their convictions, commitments, and values to see them through.

Benyamini thus reiterates Plotzker's warnings from within the profession: that the ethos inherent in the clinical approach is extremely dangerous for a nation in the constant danger that Israel is in. Like Plotzker, he too believes that the psychological approach undermines the public's values and lowers its stamina and resilience. Although psychologists may have meant to help, he insists, they weakened rather than strengthened the nation during the Gulf War.

Benyamini's criticism is given added weight by his many years of mental health work in the public domain: In addition to holding his long-standing academic position in the Psychology Department of the Hebrew University, Benyamini is one of the founders of the psychological services in the Ministry of Education; a founder of a widely used and respected hotline, Eran, which offers emergency psychological consultation; and a reserve military psychologist with experience in treating combat stress. For a man of his public record to voice the kind of doubts he did means something.

Nonetheless, whether all the moral and social ills that Benyamini and Plotzker cite can be justly laid at the doorstep of the mental health profession is certainly arguable. We should recall that both the fear and decline of social cohesion these critics complain of preceded any statements by the helping profession, and that the persons who were most fearful acted out their emotions by the asocial act of buying airplane tickets before the war even started. If some of those who stayed did so for lack of the financial means to escape, many who remained—with all their fears—were motivated by their strong sense that Israel was their home and the feeling of identification with its people and fate.

The lack of social cohesiveness for which Plotzker and Benyamini blame the mental health profession seems to have preceded rather than followed the professionals' entry into public life. Granot (1993) suggests that many of the activities undertaken by the helping professions during the war, including the services they proffered to the people who were evacuated from their homes in the wake of the missile strikes, could have been rendered just as well by a warm neighbor or friend. But this is skirting the problem.

The threat of gas and chemical attack generally cut people off from all but their closest family and friends. In this, the Gulf War was very different from the wars to which Israelis had been accustomed as well as from civil disasters in which large-scale destruction generally elicits benevolent and helping behaviors. During the Gulf War, many apartment buildings and neighborhoods in the high-risk areas were half empty as people sought refuge elsewhere, while those who stayed were, in a sense, imprisoned in their homes and their sealed rooms. Most people, especially those who had children to protect and work to cope with, were not in a position to extend much help and had no one to go to for the kind of help that they sought in the media and over the hotlines. Moreover, with the threat so amorphous and so new, it really was very difficult for people to know what to do. Avenues of active coping were also limited by the emergency routine and the possibilities at hand. People had no precedents on which to draw. And the government did not provide adequate leadership.

## MEETING A NEED

In great measure, the professionals met a real need. According to data reported in a study by Cohen et al. (1992), most (69%) of the mental health items broadcast during the war were broadcast during the first two most tense and confusing weeks, but as the public became habituated, radio preoccupation with mental health matters declined. The number and range of mental health topics discussed decreased; the number of experts who were called in declined; high-powered psychiatrists, who had initially been popular talk-show guests, disappeared from the air, leaving the field to the psychologists and educators who occupied it in ordinary times; and the bulk (67%) of the mental health issues were moved from daytime and late evening to the wee hours of the night, between midnight and 3 a.m.

Although, as Cohen and his colleagues note, the same downplaying did not occur in the newspapers, we may question whether the professionals really did do as much harm as some claimed. As we saw in Chapter 2, the vast majority of the public coped adequately. For all the legitimization of fear and encouragement of expression, people kept their fears under control, and there was no mass panic. If people were at times inconsiderate of others and unhelpful, we can ask whether their detachment was caused by the psychological advice that was given or by their isolation in their homes and sealed rooms. Nor does the public seem to believe that the professionals' enthusiasm did them much harm. A survey carried out by a consumer research agency several months after the war (Raviv, cited by Klingman, in press) found that over 40% reported that the psychological advice had helped and that less than 3% found it disturbing.

What can be said is that the public activities of the mental health professionals during the war were largely spontaneous and met a variety of needs. These, according to Professor Haim Granot (1993), dean of Bar Ilan University School of Social Work and former adviser to Israel's Civil Defense Forces, included the need to alleviate their own anxiety and the wish for self-promotion. But they also included the public's needs for information and leadership, which were not being met by the political establishment.

# References

Amcha. (1991). *Report.* National Israeli Center for Psychosocial Support of Survivors of the Holocaust and the Second Generation.

American Psychiatric Association. (1987). *Diagnostic and statistical manual of mental disorders (DMS-III-R)* (3rd ed., revised). Washington, DC: Author.

Antonovsky, A., Maoz, B., Dowty, N., & Wijsenbeek, H. (1971). Twenty-five years later: A limited study of sequelae of the concentration camp experience. *Social Psychiatry, 6,* 186–193.

Archibald, H., & Tuddenham, R. (1965). Persistent stress reactions after combat: A twenty-year follow-up. *Archives of General Psychiatry, 12,* 475–481.

Avidar, T. (1973, October 16). Women's liberation disappeared. *Ma'ariv,* p. 8.

Ayalon, O. (1983). *Precarious balance.* Tel-Aviv: Sifriat Hapoalim.

Ayalon, O. (1991). The professional's contribution in the sealed room to understanding and helping children and families in stressful situation. *Sihot, 5,* 8–13.

Ayalon, O., & Zimrin, H. (1990). *Painful childhood—A second look at child abuse.* Tel-Aviv: Sifriat Hapoalim.

Bachar, E. (1991). It is permissible to be anxious, but also to feel good. *Sihot, 5,* 13–14.

Bandura, A. (1977). Self-efficacy: Towards a unifying theory of behavioral change. *Psychological Review, 84,* 191–215.

Bandura, A. (1982). Self-efficacy mechanism in human agency. *American Psychologist, 37,* 122–147.

Barnett, R., Biener, L., & Baruch, G. K. (Eds.). (1987). *Gender and stress.* New York: Free Press.

Barocas, H., & Barocas, C. (1979). Wounds of the fathers: The next generation of Holocaust victims. *International Review Psychoanalysis, 5,* 331–341.

Bar-Yosef, R., & Padan-Eisenstark, D. (1977). Role system under stress: Sex-roles in war. *Social Problems, 25,* 135–145.

Bar-Yoseph, Y. (1991, January 30). I'm sick and tired of this mask. *Ma'ariv,* p. 1.

Barzilai, A. (1991). *Methods of working with residents of an old aged home: A social worker's personal account.* Unpublished manuscript, Tel Aviv University, School of Social Work.

Beigel, A., & Berren, M. R. (1985). Human induced disasters. *Psychiatric Annals, 15,* 143–150.

Bell, B. (1978). Disaster impact and response: Overcoming the Thousand Natural Shocks. *Gerontologist, 18,* 531–539.

Ben-David, A., & Lavee, Y. (1992). Families in the sealed room: Interaction patterns of Israeli families during SCUD missile attacks. *Family Process, 31,* 35–44.

Bendor, A., Gelkopf, M., & Sigal, M. (1993). Insanity and war: The Gulf War and the psychiatric institution. *American Journal of Psychotherapy, 47*(3), 424–442.

235

Bendor, A., Sigal, M., & Gelkopf, M. (1994). Schizophrenic inpatients and the chemical war threat. *Journal of Nervous and Mental Disease, 182*(2), 114–116.

Bennet, G. (1970). Bristol floods 1968: Controlled survey of effects in health of local community disaster. *British Medical Journal, 3,* 454–458.

Ben Yakar, M. (1991, April). *Treating evacuees in the Gulf War: Clinical lessons.* Paper presented at a conference held in Tel Aviv University, School of Social Work.

Ben-Zur, H., & Zeidner, M. (1991). Anxiety and bodily symptoms under threat of missile attack: The Israeli scene. *Anxiety Research, 4,* 35–44.

Bergman, Z. (1991). Forced intimacy—Israeli families in the Gulf War. *Sihot, 5,* Special Issue, 15–18.

Bergmann, M., & Jacoby, M. E. (1982). *Generations of the Holocaust.* New York: Basic Books.

Berman, E. (1985). *Trauma deepens trauma.* A lecture presented at the Annual Conference of the Israeli Association of Psychotherapists.

Blank, A. S. (1985). Irrational reactions to posttraumatic stress disorder and Vietnam veterans. In S. M. Sonneberg, A. S. Blank, & T. A. Talbott (Eds.), *The trauma of the war: Stress and recovery in Vietnam veterans.* Washington, DC: American Psychiatric Press.

Bleich, A., Dycian, A., Koslovsky, M., Solomon, Z., & Weiner, M. (1992). Psychiatric implications of missile attacks on civilian population. *Journal of the American Medical Association, 268,* 613–615.

Bleuler, E. (1950). *Dementia praecox or the group of schizophrenias.* New York: International Universities Press.

Bolin, R., & Klenow, D. J. (1982–1983). Response of the elderly to disaster: An age-stratified analysis. *International Journal of Aging and Human Development, 16,* 283–296.

Bordman, F. (1944). Child psychiatry in wartime Britain. *Journal of Educational Psychology, 35,* 293–301.

Borkan, J., & Reis, S. (1991). Letter to the Editor. *The New England Journal of Medicine, 325,* 583.

Borus, J. F. (1973). Re-entry II: "Making it" back to the States. *American Journal of Psychiatry, 130,* 850–854.

Boss, P., McCubbin, H. I., & Lester, G. (1979). The corporate executive wife's coping patterns in response to routine husband–father absence. *Family Process, 18,* 79–86.

Braker, I., & Gilad, Z. (1991). *Help seeking during the Gulf War: Social work observations.* Unpublished manuscript. Sheba Medical Center.

Brander, T. (1943). Psychiatric observations among Finnish children during the Russo-Finnish War of 1939–1940. *Nervous Child, 2,* 313–319.

Breznitz, S. (1992). *Memory fields.* New York: Knopf.

Brickman, P., Rabinowitz, V. C., Karuza, J., Coates, D., & Kidder, L. (1982). Modes of helping. *American Psychologist, 37,* 368–389.

Bromet, E., Schulberg, H. C., & Dunn, L. (1982). Reactions of psychiatric patients to the Three Mile Island nuclear accident. *Archives of General Psychiatry, 39,* 725–730.

Burgess, A. W., & Halmstrom, C. C. (1974). Rape trauma syndrome. *American Journal of Psychiatry, 131,* 981–986.

Burke, J. D., Jr., Borus, J. F., Burns, B. J., Millstein, K. H., & Beasley, M. C. (1982). Changes in children's behavior after a natural disaster. *American Journal of Psychiatry, 139,* 1010–1014.

Burke, J. D., Jr., Moccia, P., Borus, J. F., & Burns, B. J. (1986). Emotional distress in fifth-grade children ten months after a natural disaster. *Journal of American Academy of Child Psychiatry, 25,* 536–541.

Carmeli, A., Mevorach, L., Leiberman, N., Taubman, A., Kahanovitz, S., & Navon, D.

(1992, August). *The Gulf War: The home front in a test of crisis*. Final report. Department of Behavioral Sciences, Israel Defense Forces.

Central Bureau of Statistics. (1992). *Statistical abstract of Israel*. Jerusalem: Authors.

Chen, S. (1991, January 31). After the war we'll meet at the rabbinate. *Yediot Aharonot*, p. 31.

Chen, Y. (1991, February 12). Rehabilitation with hands tied. *Ha'aretz*, p. 3b.

Chimienti, G., Nasr, J. A., & Khalifeth, I. (1989). Children's reactions to war-related stress: Affective symptoms and behavior problems. *Social Psychiatry and Psychiatric Epidemiology*, *24*, 282–287.

Chodoff, P. (1986). Survivors of the Nazi Holocaust. In R. Moos (Ed.), *Coping with life crisis* (pp. 407–415). New York: Plenum Press.

Christenson, R. M., Walker, J. L., Ross, D. R., & Maltbie, A. A. (1981). Reactivation of traumatic conflicts. *American Journal of Psychiatry*, *138*, 984–985.

Cohen, A., Brog, A., Cheffer, C., Paz, U., Raviv, T., & Witztum, E. (1992, May). *Israelis in sealed rooms: Mental health and the mass media during the Gulf War*. Paper presented at the Annual Convention of the International Communication Association, Miami.

Cohen, A., & Dotan, J. (1976). Communication in the family as a function of stress during war and peace. *Journal of Marriage and the Family*, *38*, 141–147.

Coleman, Y. C., Butcher, Y. N., & Carson, R. C. (1980). *Abnormal psychology and modern life*. Illinois: Scott, Foresman & Co.

Collins, A. (1985). Interaction of sex-related psychological characteristics and psychoneuroendocrine stress responses. *Sex Roles*, *12*, 1219–1230.

Cowan, D. L., & Murphy, S. A. (1985). Identification of postdisaster bereavement risk predictors. *Nursing Research*, *34*, 71–75.

Danenberg, H. O., Lerman, Y., Steinlauf, S., Salomon, A., Zisman, D., Atsmon, J., & Slater, P. E. (1991). Mortality in Israel during the Persian Gulf War—Initial observations. *Israel Journal of Medical Science*, *27*, 627–630.

Danieli, Y. (1980). Families of survivors of the Nazi Holocaust: Some long- and short-term effects. In N. Milgram (Ed.), *Psychological stress and adjustment in time of war and peace*. Washington, DC: Hemisphere.

Danieli, Y. (1981). The aging Holocaust survivor: On the achievement of integration in aging survivors of the Nazi Holocaust. *Journal of Geriatric Psychiatry*, *14*, 191–209.

Dankner, A., Levy, A., & Maiberg, R. (1991). *Three in the sealed room*. Israel: Kineret.

Dasberg, H. (1987). Psychological distress of Holocaust survivors and their offspring in Israel, forty years later: A review. *Israel Journal of Psychiatry and Related Sciences*, *24*, 243–256.

Derfner, L. (1991, February 14). The view from the city hall. *The Jerusalem Report*, p. 17.

Derogatis, L. R. (1977). *The SCL-90-R manual I: Scoring, administration, and procedures for the SCL-90*. Baltimore: Johns Hopkins University, School of Medicine.

Despert, J. L. (1942). *Preliminary report on children's reactions to the war including a critical survey of the literature*. New York: Cornell University Medical College.

Dohrenwend, B. S., & Dohrenwend, B. P. (1969). *Social Status and Psychological Disorder: A Causal Inquiry*. New York: Wiley.

Dohrenwend, B. S., & Dohrenwend, B. P. (1974). *Stressful life events: Their nature and effects*. New York: Wiley.

Dohrenwend, B. S., & Dohrenwend, B. P. (1976). Sex differences and psychiatric disorders. *American Journal of Sociology*, *81*, 1447–1472.

Dohrenwend, B. P., Levav, I., Shrout, P. E., Schwartz, S., Naveh, G., Link, B. G., Skodol, A. E., & Stueve, A. (1992). Socioeconomic status and psychiatric disorders: The causation-selection issue. *Science*, *255*, 946–952.

Dolev, A. (1992, January.10). The great escape from the A region. *The Jerusalem Post City Lights Section*, p. 3.

Dollard, J., Doob, M., Mowrer, O., & Sears, R. (1939). *Frustration and aggression*. New Haven, CT: Yale University Press.

Dor-Shav, N. K. (1978). On the long-range effects of concentration camp internment of Nazi victims: Twenty-five years later. *Journal of Consulting and Clinical Psychology, 46,* 1–11.

Dotan, J., & Cohen, A. (1976). Mass media use in the family during war and peace. Israel 1973–1974. *Communication Research, 3,* 393–402.

Drabek, T. E. (1986). *Human system responses to disaster: An inventory of sociological findings*. New York: Springer-Verlag.

Earls, F., Smith, E., Reich, W., & Jung, K. G. (1988). Investigating psychopathological consequences of a disaster in children: A pilot study incorporating a structured diagnostic approach. *Journal of the American Academy of Child Adolescent Psychiatry, 27,* 90–95.

Eitinger, L. (1965). *Concentration camp survivors in Norway and Israel*. New York: Humanities Press.

Eitinger, L. (1980). The Concentration Camp Syndrome and its late sequelae. In J. Dimsdale (Ed.), *Survivors, victims and perpetrators*. Washington, DC: Hemisphere.

Eitinger, L., & Askevold, F. (1968). Psychiatric aspects. In A. Stroem (Ed.), *Norwegian concentration camp survivors* (pp. 45–84). Oslo: Humanities Press.

Epstein, S. (1983). Natural healing processes of the mind: Graded stress inoculation as an inherent coping mechanism. In D. Michenbaum & M. Yarenko (Eds.), *Stress reduction and prevention*. New York: Plenum Press.

Esroni, G. (1991, June). *A survey of the Naval Headquarters in an emergency*. Technical Report. Research Section, Behavioral Sciences Branch, Israel Navy.

Eth, S., & Pynoos, R. S. (1985). Developmental perspective on psychic trauma in childhood. In C. R. Figley (Ed.), *Trauma and its wake* (pp. 36–52). New York: Brunner/Mazel.

Everly, G. S. (1989). *The clinical guide to the treatment of human stress response*. New York: Plenum Press.

Everly, G. S., & Humphry, J. (1980). Perceived dimensions of stress responsiveness in male and female students. *Health Education, 11,* 38–39.

Eysenck, H. J. (1983). Personality as a fundamental concept in scientific psychology. *Austrian Journal of Psychology, 35,* 289–304.

Felldman, B. (1991, February). Evacuee: I'm not working, smoke packs of cigarettes, my head is empty. *Hadashot*, p. 9.

Fields, R. M. (1980). Victims of terrorism: The effects of prolonged stress. *Evaluation and Stress*, Special Issue, 76–83.

Figley, C. R. (1978). Psychological adjustment among Vietnam veterans: An overview of the research. In C. R. Figley (Ed.), *Stress disorders among Vietnam veterans: Theory, research, and treatment* (pp. 57–70). New York: Brunner/Mazel.

Frederick, C. J. (1980). Effects of natural vs. human-induced violence. *Evaluation and Change*, Special Issue, 71–75.

Frederick, C., & Pynoos, R. S. (1988). *Child Post-Traumatic Stress Reaction Index*. Los Angeles: UCLA Neuropsychiatric Institute and Hospital.

Freud, A., & Burlingham, D. T. (1943). *War and children*. New York: Medical War Books.

Gal, N. (1991, January 24). He gets on my nerves. *Yediot Aharonot*, p. 7.

Gal, R. (1991, March). *The Home front: An assessment*. Presented at the Conference of the Israeli Institute for Military Research.

Gal, R. (1992). *Stress reactions in Israel to the missile attacks during the Gulf War.* Israel Institute of Military Studies, Israel.

Gal, R., & Lazarus, R. S. (1975). The role of activity in anticipating and confronting stressful situations. *Journal of Human Stress, 1,* 4–21.

Galili, N. (1991, February 24). Now we're allowed to be afraid. *Ha'aretz,* p. 3b.

Garbarino, J., Kostelny, K., & Dubrow, K. (1991). *No place to be a child.* Toronto: Lexington Books.

Gelkopf, M., Ben-Dor, A., & Sigal, M. (in preparation). Hospital at war: The impact of the Gulf War on mental inpatients in Israel.

Gelles, R. J. (1981). *Family violence.* Beverly Hills, CA: Sage.

Gelles, R. J. (1983). An exchange/social control theory. In D. Finkelhor, R. J. Gelles, G. T. Hotaling, & M. A. Straus (Eds.), *The dark side of families: Current family violence research.* Beverly Hills, CA: Sage.

Gelles, R. J. (1985). Family violence. *Annual Review of Sociology, 11,* 347–367.

Gibbs, M. S. (1989). Factors in the victim that mediate between disaster and psychopathology: A review. *Journal of Traumatic Stress, 2*(4), 489–514.

Gilligan, C. (1982). *In a different voice.* Cambridge, MA: Harvard University Press.

Gleser, G. C., Green, B. L., & Winget, C. (1981). *Prolonged psychological effects of disaster: A study of Bufflo Creek.* New York: Academic Press.

Gove, W. R. (1972). The relationship between sex roles, marital status and mental illness. *Social Forces, 51,* 34–44.

Gove, W. R. (1979). Sex differences in the epidemiology of mental disorder: Evidence and explanation. In E. Gomberg & V. Franks (Eds.), *Gender-disordered behavior.* New York: Brunner/Mazel.

Gove, W. R., & Tudor, J. F. (1973). Adult sex roles and mental illness. *American Journal of Sociology, 78,* 812–835.

Granot, H. (1993). Over reacting and mis-reacting during the Gulf War. *Hevra Verevaha, 13*(3), 301–307.

Greenbaum, C., Erlich, C., & Toubiana, Y. (1992, January). *Sex differences in delayed effects of exposure to Gulf War stress by Israeli city settler children.* Paper presented at the Ministry of Education Conference on Stress Reactions in Children in the Gulf War, Ramat Gan.

Grinblatt, J. (1991, March 3). 9000 apartments damaged by missiles in the Gush Dan area: Only two-thirds of them repaired. *Ha'aretz,* p. 5a.

Grisaru, N., Paronsky, A., Zabow, A., & Belmaker, R. H. (1993). The effect of life-threatening war stress on an acute psychiatric ward. *Stress Medicine, 9*(3), 141–143.

Guri, S. (1992, January). Interview, personal communication.

Hantman, S. (1992). *The effect of prior traumatic experience on anxiety symptoms in the aged during the Gulf War.* Unpublished master's thesis, Tel-Aviv University.

Har-Even, S. (1991, January 21). Not on fear alone. *Yediot Aharonot,* p. 27.

Helson, H. (1964). *Adaptation level theory: The experimental and systematic approach to behavior.* New York: Harper & Row.

Hill, R. (1949). *Families under stress.* New York: Harper & Row.

Himmelfarb, S., & Murrel, S. A. (1983). Reliability and validity of five mental health scales in older persons. *Journal of Gerontology, 38,* 333–339.

Himmelfarb, S., & Murrel, S. A. (1984). The prevalence and correlates of anxiety symptoms in older adults. *Journal of Psychology, 116,* 159–167.

Hinkle, L. E. J. (1974). The effect of exposure to cultural change, social change and changes in interpersonal relationships on health. In B. S. Dohrenwend & B. P. Dohrenwend (Eds.), *Stressful life events: Their nature and effects.* New York: Wiley.

Hobfoll, S., Lomranz, J., Eyal, N., Bridges, A., & Tzemach, M. (1989). Pulse of a nation:

Depressive mood reactions of Israelis to the Israel–Lebanon War. *Journal of Personality and Social Psychology, 56,* 1002–1012.

Hobfoll, S., & London, P. (1986). The relationship of self concept and social support to emotional distress among women during war. *Journal of Social and Clinical Psychology, 4,* 189–203.

Hoffman, M. A., Levy-Shiff, R., Solberg, S. C., & Zarizki, J. (1992). The impact of stress and coping: Developmental changes in the transition to adolescence. *Journal of Youth and Adolescence, 27,* 39–45.

Hoiberg, A., McCaughey, B. G. (1984). The traumatic after-effects of collision at sea. *American Journal of Psychiatry, 141,* 70–74.

Holmes, T. H., & Rahe, R. H. (1967). The Social Readjustment Scale. *Journal of Psychosomatic Research, 11,* 213–218.

Horowitz, M. H., Wilner, N., & Alvarez, W. (1979). Impact of Event Scale: A measure of subjective stress. *Psychological Medicine, 42,* 209–218.

Huminer, D., Pitlik, S. D., Katz, A., Metzker, A., & David, M. (1991). Untoward effects of gas masks during the Persian Gulf War. *New England Journal of Medicine, 325,* 582.

Hunter, E. (1978). The Vietnam POW veteran: Immediate and long-term. In C. R. Figley (Ed.), *Stress disorders among Vietnam veterans: Theory, research and treatment.* New York: Brunner/Mazel.

IDF Mental Health Department. (1991, January). Emotional stress of a threatened population and its treatment. Internal memo.

Israelshvili, M. (1992, January). *The effect of the Gulf War on the feelings of youth and their willingness to serve in the Israel Defense Forces.* Unpublished paper, School of Education, Tel-Aviv University.

Itskovitz, R., & Strauss, H. (1982). *The Bar-Ilan Picture Test for Children* (revised edition). Copenhagen: Denmark's Pedagogical Institute Test Service.

Janis, I. L. (1951). *Air war and emotional distress.* New York: McGraw-Hill.

Janis, I. L. (1971). *Stress and frustration.* New York: Harcourt Brace Jovanovich.

Janoff-Bullman, R. (1989). Assumptive worlds and the stress of traumatic events: Applications of the schema construct. *Social Cognition, 7,* 113–136.

Janoff-Bullman, R., & Frieze, I. H. (1987). The role of gender in reaction to criminal victimization. In R. C. Barnett, L. Beienr, & G. K. Baruch (Eds.), *Gender and stress* (pp. 159–184). New York: Free Press.

Kachlili, R. (1991, January 23). Don't worry kids, we're all afraid. *Hadashot,* p. 20.

Kaffman, M. (1977). Kibbutz civilian population under war stress. *British Journal of Psychiatry, 30,* 489–494.

Kaplan, Z., Kron, S., Lichtenberg, P., Solomon, Z., & Bleich, A. (1992). Military mental health in the Gulf War: The experience of the central clinic of the IDF. *Israel Journal of Psychiatry and Related Sciences, 29,* 7–13.

Kaplan, Z., Singer, Y., Lichtenberg, P., Solomon, Z., & Bleich, A. (1992). PTSD in Israel during the Gulf War. *Israel Journal of Psychiatry and Related Sciences, 29,* 14–21.

Katzanelson, E. (1991, January 23). Helping your kids get back on track. *Ma'ariv,* p. 7.

Katzman, A. (1991, March 3). Let's talk about it: Interview with Kalman Benyamimi. *Ha'aretz,* pp. 16–17.

Kedem, M. (1991a, February 2). Aviva Gruendland returns to her destroyed home: I'm still looking for my husband. *Hadashot,* p. 19.

Kedem, M. (1991b, February 10). Don't cry grandpa. As long as nobody died. We'll build a new house. *Hadashot,* p. 6.

Keinan, G. (1979). *The effects of personality and training variables on the experiences, stress and quality of performance in situations where physical integrity is threatened.* Unpublished doctoral dissertation, Tel-Aviv University.

Kersenty, E., Shemer, J., Alshech, I., Cojocaru, B., Moscowitz, M., Shapiro, Y., & Danon, Y. L. (1991). Medical aspects of the Iraqi missile attacks on Israel. *Israel Journal of Medical Science, 27,* 603–607.

Kessler, R. C., & Maleod, J. D. (1984). Sex differences in vulnerability to undesirable life events. *American Sociological Review, 49,* 620–631.

Kinston, W., & Rosser, R. (1974). Disaster: Effects on mental and physical health. *Journal of Psychosomatic Response, 18,* 437–456.

Klausner, A. (1991, February 2). Children of the Scud. *Journal of Medicine and Family Health,* pp. 1–14.

Klingman, A. (1992). Stress reactions of Israeli youth during the Gulf War: A quantitative study. *Professional Psychology: Research Practice, 23*(6), 521–527.

Klingman, A., Sagi, A., & Raviv, A. (1993). The effect of war on Israeli children. In L. A. Leavitt & N. A. Fox (Eds.), *Psychological effects of war and violence on children* (pp. 75–92). Hillsdale, NJ: Erlbaum.

Klonoff, E. A. (1983). A star is born: Psychologists and the media. *Professional Psychology: Research and Practice, 14*(6), 847–854.

Kluznik, J. C., Speed, N., van Valkenburg, C., & Margraw, R. (1986). Forty-year follow-up of United States' prisoners of war. *American Journal of Psychiatry, 143,* 1443–1446.

Knoller, J. (1991a, February 20). The Pnimiot didn't give shelter. *Ha'aretz,* p. 2b.

Knoller, J. (1991b, January 22). Psychologists advise legitimization of children's anxieties. Interview with Bina Weiler. *Ha'aretz,* p. 6a.

Kol Israel, IBS (1991, January 17).

Kristal, L. (1978). Bruxism: An anxiety response to environmental stress. In C. D. Spielberger, & I. G. Sarason (Eds.), *Stress and anxiety* (vol. 5). Washington, DC: Hemisphere.

Kroll, A. (1991, February 20). Good days for the paranoids. *Ha'aretz,* p. 4b.

Krystal, H. (1981). The aging survivor of the Holocaust: Integration and self healing in post-traumatic states. *Journal of Geriatric Psychiatry, 14,* 165–189.

Kulka, R. A., Schlenger, W. E., Fairbank, J. A., Hough, R. L., Jordan, B. K., Marmar, C. R., & Weiss, O. S. (1988). *Contractual report of findings from the National Vietnam Veterans Readjustment Study.* Research Triangle Park, NC: Research Triangle Institute.

Lacey. G. N. (1972). Observations on Aberfan. *Journal of Psychosomatic Research, 16,* 257–260.

Laufer, R. S., Frey-Wouters, E., & Gallops, M. S. (1985). Traumatic stressors in the Vietnam War and posttraumatic stress disorder. In C. R. Figley (Ed.), *Trauma and its wake* (vol. 1, pp. 73–89). New York: Brunner/Mazel.

Lavee, Y., & Ben-David, A. (1993). Families under war: Stress and strains of Israeli families during the Gulf War. *Journal of Traumatic Stress, 6*(2), 945–951.

Lavie, D. (1991, January 23). The children who stayed at home. *Ma'ariv,* p. 1.

Lavie, J. (1991, January 22). In praise of anxiety. *Ha'aretz,* p. 7.

Lavie, P., Amit, Y., Epstein, R., & Tzischinsky, O. (1992, June). *Children sleep under the threat of the Scud.* Paper presented at the Annual Meeting of the Association of Sleep Research, Phoenix, Arizona.

Lavie, P., Carmeli, A., Mevorach, L., & Liberman, N. (1991). Sleeping under the threat of the Scud: War-related environmental insomnia. *Israel Journal of Medical Science, 27,* 681–686.

Lazarus, R. S. (1986). The psychology of stress and coping. In C. D. Spielberger & I. C. Sarason (Eds.), *Stress and anxiety, Vol. 10* (pp. 399–418). Washington, DC: Hemisphere.

Lazarus, R. S., & Folkman, S. (1984). *Stress, appraisal and coping.* New York: Springer-Verlag.

Leon, G. R., Butcher, J. N., Kleinman, M., Goldberg, K., & Almagor, M. (1981). Survivors of the Holocaust and their children: Current status and adjustment. *Journal of Personality and Social Psychology, 41,* 503–506.

Lev-Ari, R., & Bostan, D. (1991, June). After the blow: Abused wives coping with family violence. Tel Aviv, Israel.

Levin, Y., Barkai, R., Levkowitch, Y., Weiser, M., Levy, A., & Neumann, M. *Psychological coping styles of schizophrenic inpatients and nursing staff members with the chemical and nuclear threat of the 1991 Gulf War.* In preparation.

Levy, A. (1991). Air-raid in a closed department: Double entry. *Sihot, 5,* Special Issue, 20–21.

Levy, S. (1991a, February 1). Support for the government: Just like the Six Day War. *Ma'ariv,* pp. 7–8.

Levy, S. (1991b, February). *Morale during the Gulf War.* Lecture presented at the Israeli Institute for Military Studies, Zichron Ya'acov.

Leiblich, A. (1983). Between strength and toughness. In S. Breznitz (Ed.), *Stress in Israel.* New York: Van Nostrand Reinhold.

Lieblich, A. (1988). *Tin soldiers on Jerusalem Beach.* Tel-Aviv: Schocken.

Lindeman, E. (1944). Symptomatology and management of acute grief. *American Journal of Psychiatry, 101,* 141–148.

Livni, N. (1991, January 20). Parents, fear not fear. *Hadashot,* p. 20.

Lomranz, J. (1990). Long-term adaptation to traumatic stress in light of adult development and aging perspectives. In M. A. P. Stephens, J. H. Crowther, S. Hobfoll, & D. L. Tennebaum (Eds.), *Stress and coping in later life families* (pp. 99–121). Washington, DC: Hemisphere.

Lomranz, J., & Eyal, N. (1994). Longitudinal study of depressive moods of men and women in different age groups during the Gulf War. In J. Lomranz & G. Naveh (Eds.), *Trauma and old age: Coping with the stress of the Gulf War* (pp. 13–29). Jerusalem: JDC-Brookdale Institute of Gerontology.

Lomerantz, J., Shmotkin, D., Zchovoi, A., & Rosenberg, E. (1985). Time orientation in Nazi concentration camps: Forty years after. *American Journal of Orthopsychiatry, 55,* 230–236.

Lubin, B. (1967). *Depression Adjective Checklist: Manual.* San Diego, CA: Educational and Industrial Services.

Luria, O. (1991, June). *Coping of air force soldiers in the central region during the first weeks of the war.* Technical Report. Research Section, Psychology Branch, Israel Air Force.

McCubbin, H. I., & Patterson, J. M. (1983). The family stress process: The double ABCX model of adjustment and adaptation. In H. I. McCubbin, M. Sussman, & J. Patterson (Eds.), *Social stress and the family* (pp. 7–37). New York: Haworth Press.

McFarlane, A. C., Policansky, S., & Irwin, C. P. (1987). A longitudinal study of the psychological morbidity in children due to a natural disaster. *Psychological Medicine, 17,* 727–738.

McGrath, J. E. (1970). Setting measures and theses: An integrative review of some research of social and psychological factors in stress. In J. E. McGrath (Ed.), *Social and psychological factors in stress* (pp. 558–596). New York: Holt, Rinehart & Winston.

Meichenbaum, D. (1985). *Stress inoculation training.* New York: Pergamon Press.

Meidan, A. (1991, February 5). Holocaust survivors and the gas masks. *Hadashot,* pp. 20–21.

Meisel, S. R., Kutz, I., Dayan, K. I., Pauzner, H., Chetboun, I., Arbel, Y., & David, D. (1991). Effect of the Iraqi missile war on incidence of acute myocardial infarction and sudden death in Israeli civilians. *Lancet, 338,* 660–661.

Meisels, R. (1991). *Psychological aid to the civilian population before and during a non-conventional war.* Unpublished manuscript.

Melamed, Y., Elizur, A., Solomon, Z., & Schur, H. (in preparation). *Mental patients' functioning during the Gulf War.*

Melick, M. E., & Logue, J. N. (1985–1986). The effect of disaster on the health and well-being of older women. *International Journal of Aging and Human Development, 21,* 27–38.

Mendler, N. (1991, January 21). We could have died. *Ha'aretz,* p. 2b.

Middleton, W., & Raphael, B. (1990). Consultation in disasters. *International Journal of Mental Health, 19,* 109–120.

Mikulincer, M., Solomon, Z., & Benbenishty, R. (1988). Battle events, acute CSR and long-term psychological sequelae of war. *Journal of Anxiety Disorders, 2*(2) 121–133.

Milgram, N. A. (1978). Psychological stress and adjustment in time of war and peace: The Israeli experience as presented in two conferences. *Israel Annals of Psychiatry and Related Disciplines, 16,* 327–338.

Milgram, N. A. (1982). War-related stress in Israeli children and youth. In L. Goldberg & S. Breznitz (Eds.), *Handbook of Stress: Theoretical and Clinical Aspects* (pp. 656–676). New York: Free Press.

Milgram, N. A., & Miller, M. S. (1973). *The influence of extended shelling on the levels of manifest anxiety and autonomy of children.* Unpublished manuscript, Bar-Ilan University.

Milgram, N. A., Toubiana, Y. H., Klingman, A., & Raviv, A. (1988). Situational exposure and personal loss in children's acute and chronic stress reactions to a school-bus disaster. *Journal of Traumatic Stress, 1,* 339–352.

Milgram, R. M., & Milgram, N. A. (1976). The effect of the Yom Kippur War on anxiety level in Israeli children. *Journal of Psychology, 94,* 107–113.

Miller, R. G. (1981). *Simultaneous statistical inference.* New York: Springer-Verlag.

Mintz, M. (1992, January). *A comparison between children in two areas following the Gulf War.* Paper presented at the Ministry of Education Conference on Stress Reactions of Children in the Gulf War, Ramat Gan.

Miron, M. (1991, February 1). The impossible to recreate. *Ha'aretz,* p. 5b.

Murphy, J. M., Sobol, A. M., Neff, R. K., Olivier, D. C., & Leighton, A. H. (1984). Stability and prevalence: Depression and anxiety disorders. *Archives of General Psychiatry, 41,* 990–997.

Nader, K., Pynoos, R. S., Fairbanks, L., & Fredrick, C. (1990). Children's PTSD reactions one year after a sniper attack at their school. *American Journal of Psychiatry, 147*(11), 1526–1530.

Nadler, A. (1983). Social psychology and social issues: Research and theory on help seeking and help receiving in applied settings. In A. Nadler et al. (Eds.), *New directions in helping* (vol. 3). New York: Academic Press.

Nadler, A. (1989). Forty years later: Long-term consequences of massive traumatization as manifested by Holocaust survivors from the city and the kibbutz. *Journal of Consulting and Clinical Psychology, 57,* 287–293.

Namir, D. (1991, January 25). Should a child be awakened because of nightmares? A psychiatrist answers parents' questions. *Yediot Aharonot,* p. 10.

Nardi, C. (1992, January). Interview, personal communication.

Nasjleti, M. (1980). Suffering in silence: The male incest victim. *Child Welfare, 59,* 271.

Navon, D. (1992, August). Public fear legitimization, Appendix. In A. Carmeli, L. Mevorach, N. Leiberman, A. Taubman, S. Kahanovitz, & D. Navon (Eds.), *The Gulf War: The home front in a test of crisis.* IDF: Department of Behavioral Sciences.

Neiderland, W. G. (1968). The problem of the survivor. In H. Krystal (Ed.), *Massive psychic trauma.* New York: International University Press.

Nevo, A. (1991, January 24). The minute they begin to call you "evacuee." *Yediot Aharonot*, p. 26.

Newman, C. J. (1976). Children of disaster: Clinical observations at Buffalo Creek. *American Journal of Psychiatry, 133*, 306–316.

Newman, E. C. (1989). Stress and the contemporary woman. In G. Everly, (Ed.), *The clinical guide to the treatment of human stress response*. New York: Plenum Press.

Nicols, B., & Czirr, R. (1986). Post-traumatic stress disorder: Hidden syndrome in elders. *Clinical Gerontologist, 5*, 417–433.

Norris, F. H., & Murrel, S. A. (1988). Prior experience as a moderator of disaster impact on anxiety symptoms in older adults. *American Journal of Community Psychology, 16*, 665–683.

Notman, M., & Nadelson, C. (1976). The rape victim: Psychodynamic consideration. *American Journal of Psychiatry, 133*, 408–412.

Noy, B. (1991). *Students' use of the open line during the emergency period of the Gulf War*. Jerusalem: Ministry of Education, Pedagogical Unit.

Noy, S. (1991). *I can not anymore*. Israel: Israel Ministry of Defense.

Omer, H. (1991). Mass casualties: The role of emergency teams. *Sihot, 5*, 48–60.

Palacios, A., Cueli, J., Camacho, J., Cleriga, R., Cuevas, J. A., & Cossof, L. (1986). The traumatic effect of mass communication in the Mexico City earthquake. *International Review of Psych-Analysis, 13*, 279–293.

Parsons, O. A., & Schneider, J. M. (1974). Locus of control in university students from Eastern and Western societies. *Journal of Consulting and Clinical Psychology, 42*, 456–461.

Pearlin, L. I. (1975). Sex role and depression. In N. Datan and L. H. Ginsberg, (Eds.), *Life-span developmental psychology: Normative life crises*. New York: Academic Press.

Pearlin, L. I., & Schooler, C. (1978). The structure of coping. *Journal of Health and Social Behavior, 19*, 2–21.

Peled, T., & Katz, E. (1974). Media functions in wartime: The Israel home front in October 1973. In J. G. Blumler & E. Katz (Eds.), *Mental health responses to mass emergencies* (pp. 3–21). New York: Brunner/Mazel.

Peleg, M. (1991, January). Interview with Colonel Hedva Almog. *Be'mahane*, p. 9.

Plotzker, S. (1991, February 2). The other side of fear. *Yediot Aharonot*, p. 27.

Pynoos, R. S., & Eth, S. (1985). Developmental perspective on psychic trauma in childhood. In C. R. Figley (Ed.), *Trauma and its wake* (vol. 2, pp. 36–52). New York: Brunner/Mazel.

Pynoos, R. S., Fredrick, C., Nader, K., Arroyo, W., Steinberg, A., Eth, S., Nunez, F., & Fairbanks, L. (1987). Life threat and post-traumatic stress in school-age children. *Archives of General Psychiatry, 44*, 1057–1063.

Quarantelli, E. L., & Dynes, R. R. (1985). Community responses to disaster. In B. J. Sowder (Ed.), *Disaster and mental health: Selected contemporary perspectives* (pp. 158–168). Rockville, MD: National Institute for Mental Health.

Rachman, S. (1990). *Fear and courage*. New York: Freeman.

Rahe, R. H. (1974). Life change and subsequent illness reports. In E. K. E. Gunderson & R. H. Rahe (Eds.), *Life stress and illness*. Springfield, IL: C. C. Thomas.

Rahe, R. H. (1988). Acute versus chronic psychological reactions to combat. *Military Medicine, 153*, 365–372.

Rahe, R. H., & Arthur, R. J. (1970). Life changes surrounding illness experience. *Journal of Psychosomatic Research, 14*, 121–123.

Randolph, L. S., & Rahe, D. S. (1979). Susceptibility and precipitating factors in depression: Sex differences and similarities. *Journal of Abnormal Psychology, 88*, 174–181.

Raviv, A., & Raviv, A. (1991). *Telephone surveys during and after the Gulf War.* Unpublished report, Tel Aviv University, Department of Psychology, Department of Statistics.

Rinat, Z. (1991, February 1). Children's homes. *Ha'aretz*, p. 5b.

Ringle-Hoffman, A. (1991, January 21). Children of the Scud. *Yediot Aharonot*, pp. 4–5.

Robinson, S., & Netanel, R. (1991). Reactions of Holocaust survivors to the Gulf War and Scud missile attacks on Israel. *Echoes of the Holocaust, 1,* 1.

Rofe, Y. (1989). *Repression and fear: A new approach to resolve the crisis in psychopathology.* New York: Hemisphere.

Rofe, Y., & Lewin, I. (1982). The effect of war environment on dreams and sleep habits. In C. D. Spielberger, I. G. Sarason, & N. A. Milgram (Eds.), *Stress and anxiety* (vol. 8). Washington, DC: Hemisphere.

Rogers, C. M., & Terry, T. (1984). Clinical interventions with boy victims of sexual abuse. In I. R. Stuart & J. G. Greer (Eds.), *Victims of sexual aggression: Treatment of children, women and men.* New York: Van Nostrand Reinhold.

Ronen, T., & Rahav, G. (1992, January). *Children's behavior problems during the Gulf War.* Paper presented at the Israeli Ministry of Education Conference on Stress Reactions of Children in the Gulf War, Ramat Gan.

Rosenbaum, M., & Ronen, T. (1992, January). *How did Israeli children and their parents cope with the threat of daily attack by Scud missiles during the Gulf War?* Paper presented at the Ministry of Education Conference on Stress Reactions of Children in the Gulf War, Ramat Gan.

Rosenthal, M., & Levy-Shiff, R. (1993). Threat of missile attacks in the Gulf War: Mothers' perceptions of young children's reactions. *American Journal of Orthopsychiatry, 63*(2), 241–254.

Rudi, D. (1991, February). *Psychologists in the Gulf War.* Lecture presented at Zikhron Ya'acov, the Center for Military Studies.

Russo, N. (1991, January 25). My spouse and I: Who won? *Ha'aretz*, p. 6.

Saffir, M., Merbaum, M., Goldberg, J., & Yinon, Y. (1977). Fear in periods of stress and calm among Israeli students. *Journal of Behavioral Therapy and Experimental Psychiatry, 8,* 5–9.

Saigh, P. (1984). Pre- and postinvasion anxiety in Lebanon. *Behavior Therapy, 15,* 185–190.

Saigh, P. (1988). Anxiety, depression and assertion across alternating intervals of stress. *Journal of Abnormal Psychology, 97,* 338–341.

Schacter, S. (1959). *The psychology of affiliation.* Palo Alto, CA: Stanford University Press.

Schlosberg, A. *Mental patients during the Gulf War.* Unpublished manuscript.

Schulberg, H. (1974). Disaster crisis theory and intervention strategies. *Omega, 5,* 77–87.

Schwarzwald, J., Weisenberg, M., Solomon, Z., & Waysman, M. (in preparation). Stress reactions of school-age children to the bombardment by Scud missiles: A one year follow-up.

Schwarzwald, J., Weisenberg, M., Waysman, M., Solomon, Z., & Klingman, A. (1993). Stress reactions of school-age children to the bombardment by Scud missiles. *Journal of Abnormal Psychology, 102*(3), 404–410.

Selye, H. (1956). *The stress of life.* New York: McGraw-Hill.

Selye, H. (1970). Stress and aging. *Journal of the American Geriatric Society, 18,* 660–681.

Shabi, A. (1991, February 1). If you're hit by a missile, it's better in Ramat Gan. *Yediot Aharonot*, p. 11.

Shaked, I. (1991, February 2). Cooking in their own juice in a pressure cooker. *Ma'ariv*, pp. 27–28.

Shalev, A. (1991a). Three comments on the war, the therapist and the possible trauma. *Sihot, 5,* 6–8.

Shalev, A. (1991b, October). *The Israeli population in the Gulf War.* Lecture presented at the 5th Annual Conference of the International Society of Traumatic Stress Studies, Washington, DC.

Shanan, J., & Shahar, O. (1983). Cognitive and personality functioning of Jewish Holocaust survivors during midlife transition in Israel. *Archives of Psychology, 135,* 275–294.

Shapira, Y., Marganitt, B., Roziner, I., Shochet, T., Bar, Y., & Shemer, J. (1991). Willingness of staff to report to their hospital duties following an unconventional missile attack: A state-wide survey. *Israel Journal of Medical Science, 27,* 704–711.

Shuval, J. T., Markus, E. J., Dotan, J. (1973). *Patterns of adjustment of Soviet immigrants to Israel.* Jerusalem: Israel Institute of Applied Social Research.

Shuval, Y. (1963). The concentration camp. In Y. Shuval (Ed.), *Immigrants on the threshold* (pp. 79–103). New York: Atherton Press.

Silver, R. L., & Wortman, C. B. (1980). Coping with undesirable life events. In J. Garber & M. E. P. Seligman (Eds.), *Human helplessness.* New York: Academic Press.

Solomon, Z. (1988). The effect of combat related posttraumatic stress disorder on the family. *Psychiatry, 51,* 323–329.

Solomon, Z. (1989a). A three-year prospective study of posttraumatic stress disorder in Israeli combat veterans. *Journal of Traumatic Stress, 2*(1), 59–73.

Solomon, Z. (1989b). Untreated combat-related PTSD—why some Israeli veterans do not seek help. *Israel Journal of Psychiatry and Related Sciences, 26,* 111–123.

Solomon, Z. (1993). *Combat stress reaction: The enduring toll of war.* New York: Plenum Press.

Solomon, Z., Benbenishty, R., & Mikulincer, M. (1988). A follow-up of Israeli casualties of combat stress reaction ("battle shock") in the 1982 Lebanon War. *British Journal of Clinical Psychology, 22,* 125–135.

Solomon, Z., Garb, R., Bleich, A., & Grupper, D. (1987). Reactivation of combat related post-traumatic stress disorder. *American Journal of Psychiatry, 144,* 51–55.

Solomon, Z., Laor, N., Weiler, D., Muller, U. F., Hadar, O., Waysman, M., Koslowsky, M., Ben Yakar, M., & Bleich, A. (1993). The psychological impact of the Gulf War: A study of acute stress in Israeli evacuees. *Archives of General Psychiatry, 50,* 320–321.

Solomon, Z., Margalit, C., Waysman, M., & Bleich, A. (1991). In the shadow of the Gulf War: Psychological distress, social support and coping among Israeli soldiers in a high-risk area. *Israel Journal of Medical Science, 27,* 673.

Solomon, Z., Mikulincer, M., & Benbenishty, R. (1989a). Combat stress reaction: Clinical manifestations and correlates. *Military Psychology, 1*(1), 35–47.

Solomon, Z., Mikulincer, M., & Benbenishty, R. (1989b). Locus of control and combat-related posttraumatic stress disorder: the intervening role of battle intensity, threat appraisal, and coping. *British Journal of Clinical Psychology, 28,* 131–144.

Solomon, Z., Mikulincer, M., & Hobfoll, S. (1987). Objective versus subjective measurement of stress and social support: The case of combat-related reactions. *Journal of Consulting and Clinical Psychology, 55,* 577–583.

Solomon, Z., Mikulincer, M., & Jacob, B. R. (1987). Exposure to recurrent combat stress: Combat stress reaction among Israeli soldiers in the 1982 Lebanon War. *Psychological Medicine, 17,* 433–440.

Solomon, Z., Noy, S., & Bar-On, R. (1986). Risk factors in combat stress reaction—a study of Israeli soldiers in the 1982 Lebanon War. *Israel Journal of Psychiatry and Related Science, 23,* 3–8.

Solomon, Z., Oppenheimer, B., Elizur, Y., & Waysman, M. (1990). Exposure to recurrent combat stress: Can successful coping in a second war heal combat-related PTSD from the past? *Journal of Anxiety Disorders, 4,* 141–145.

Solomon, Z., Weisenberg, M., Schwarzwald, J., & Mikulincer, M. (1987). PTSD among front-line soldiers with combat stress reactions: The 1982 Israeli experience. *American Journal of Psychiatry, 144*(4), 448–454.

Solomon, Z., Weisenberg, M., Schwarzwald, J., & Mikulincer, M. (1988). CSR and PTSD as determinants of perceived self-efficacy in battle. *Journal of Social and Clinical Psychology, 6*, 356–370.

Spielberger, C. D., Gorsuch, R. L., & Lushene, R. E. (1970). *Manual for the State-Trait Anxiety Inventory.* Palo Alto, CA: Consulting Psychologists Press.

Stern, M. (1992). Reflections on the Gulf War. *Sihot, 7*, 53–56.

Strayer, R., & Ellenhorn, L. (1975). Vietnam veterans: A study exploring adjustment patterns and attitudes. *Journal of Social Issues, 31*, 81–94.

Strobe, M. S., & Strobe, W. (1983). Who suffers more? Sex differences in depressive symptomatology: A community study. *Journal of Health and Social Behavior, 14*, 291–299.

Strumpfer, D. J. (1970). Fear and affiliation during a disaster. *Journal of Social Psychology, 82*, 263–268.

Talmon, Y., Guy, N., Mure, K., Rafes, A., & Naor, S. (1992). The Sadaam Syndrome: Acute psychotic reactions during the Gulf War. *Ha'refua, 123*, 237–240.

Terr, L. C. (1983). Chowchilla revisited: The effects of psychic trauma four years after a school-bus kidnapping. *American Journal of Psychiatry, 140*, 1543–1550.

Terr, L. C. (1985). Psychic trauma in children and adolescents. *Psychiatric Clinics of North America, 8*, 815–835.

Titchner, J. L. (1986). Post-traumatic decline: A consequence of unresolved destructive drives. In C. R. Figley (Ed.), *Trauma and its wake. 2. Traumatic stress, theory, research and intervention.* New York: Brunner/Mazel.

Titchner, J. L., & Ross, W. O. (1974). Acute or chronic stress as determinants of behavior, character, and neuroses. In S. Arieti & E. B. Brody (Eds.), *American handbook of psychiatry* (2nd ed., pp. 39–60). New York: Basic Books.

Toubiana, Y., Goldstein, I., & Hareven, D. (1992, January). *The stress reactions and interest in help in school children during and after the Gulf War.* Paper presented at the Ministry of Education Conference on Stress Reactions of Children in the Gulf War, Ramat Gan.

Trabelski, T., & Rosolio, M. (1991, January 28). Tel Aviv evacuees: Ramat Gan evacuees got better hotels, *Yediot Aharonot*, p. 12.

Vardy, D. A., Laver, Z., Zakai-Rones, Z., Klaus, S. N. (1991). Letter to the Editor. *New England Journal of Medicine, 325*, 583.

Vinokur, A., & Selzer, M. (1975). Desirable versus undesirable life events: Their relationship to stress and mental distress. *Journal of Personality and Social Psychology, 32*, 329–337.

Wallerstein, J. S., & Blakeslee, S. (1989). *Second chances: Men, women and children after divorce.* New York: Tiknor and Fields.

Weil, F. (1975). Civilians under war stress. *Psychiatric Journal of the University of Ottowa, 10*(10):53–55.

Weisenberg, M., Schwarzwald, J., Waysman, M., Solomon, Z., & Klingman, A. (1993). Coping of school-age children in the sealed room during Scud missile bombardment and post-war stress reaction. *Journal of Consulting and Clinical Psychology, 61*, 462–467.

Weissman, M., & Kelerman, G. (1977). Sex difference and the epidemiology of depression. *Archives of General Psychiatry, 34*, 98–111.

Why wasn't he called up? (1973, October 8). *Ma'ariv*, p. 4.

Woods, N., & Hulka, B. (1979). Symptom reports and illness behavior among employed women and homemakers. *Journal of Community Health, 5*, 36–45.

Yizhaki, T., Solomon, Z., & Kotler, M. (1991). The clinical picture of acute combat stress reaction among Israeli soldiers in the 1982 Lebanon War. *Military Medicine, 156*(4), 193–197.

Yule, W. (1991). Children in shipping disasters. *Journal of the Royal Society of Medicine, 84,* 12–15.

Yule, W., & Williams, R. M. (1990). Post-traumatic stress reactions in children. *Journal of Traumatic Stress, 3,* 279–295.

Zak, I. (1982). Stability and change in personality traits: Possible effects of the Yom Kippur War on Israeli youth. In C. D. Spielberger, I. G. Sarason, & N. A. Milgram (Eds.), *Stress and anxiety* (vol. 8). Washington, DC: Hemisphere.

Zaslow, M. J., & Hays, C. D. (1986). Sex differences in children's response to psychological stress: Toward a cross-context analysis. In M. E. Lamb, A. L. Brown, & B. Roggof (Eds.), *Advances in Developmental Psychology* (vol. 4, pp. 285–338). Hillsdale, NJ: Erlbaum.

Zeidner, M., & Ben-Zur, H. (1989). The Hebrew adaptation of the State-Trait Personality Inventory. In R. Schwarzer, H. M. van der Ploeg, & C. D. Spielberger (Eds.), *Advances in test anxiety research* (vol. 6, pp. 253–262). Lisse, The Netherlands: Swets & Zeitlinger.

Zeidner, M., Klingman, A., & Itskovitz, R. (1993). Children's affective reactions and coping under threat of missile attack: A semiprojective assessment procedure. *Journal of Personality Assessment, 60*(3), 435–457.

Zimran, A., & Ashkenazi, Y. J. (1991). Letter to the Editor. *New England Journal of Medicine, 325,* 583.

Ziv, A. (1975). *Empirical findings on children's reaction to war stress.* Paper presented to the First Conference on Psychological Stress and Adjustment in Time of War and Peace, Tel Aviv.

Ziv, A., & Israeli, R. (1973). Effects of bombardment on the manifest anxiety levels of children living in the kibbutz. *Journal of Consulting and Clinical Psychology, 40,* 287–291.

Ziv, A., Kruglanski, A. W., & Shulman, S. (1974). Children's psychological reactions to wartime stress. *Journal of Personality and Social Psychology, 30,* 24–30.

# Index

Flight, 8–9, 14, 32, 34, 46, 47, 116, 232. *See also* Leaving home
Follow-up, 117, 158, 159, 164–169, 179
Forced passivity, 4–5, 15, 18, 32, 35, 84
  and Holocaust survivors, 139
  *See also* Policy of restraint

Gas masks, 6, 7, 8, 9, 10, 11–12, 13, 16, 17, 18, 20, 21, 31, 36, 42
  and children, 7, 12, 74
  and illness, 53
  *See also* Protective devices
Gender difference, xvi, 18, 123
  and anxiety, 94, 96, 131
  and compliance, 93
  and coping, 84, 93, 98, 122
  and depression, 94, 95
  and fear, 93, 94
  and habituation, 93
  and protective device, 93
  role conflict, 87–92, 98–99
  and routine disruption, 94
  and sensitivities, 99–100
  and sleep disturbances, 92–93
  and somatic complaints, 94
  and wartime, 81–101, 194
  and work, 96–98
General psychiatric symptomatology, 161, 165, 169–170, 199
Gulf War stressors, vii, xvi, 1, 2, 3, 4, 5–11, 16, 18–21, 58–59, 61–62, 65, 72
  and the elderly, 133, 136
  and gender, 194
  and mental health professionals, 213–215, 225
  and soldiers, 192–194

Habituation, viii–ix, xvi, 23, 26, 33, 34, 36, 37, 39, 44, 47, 50, 52, 54, 93, 109, 111–112, 113, 128. *See also* Accommodation; Adaptation

Help seeking, 50–51, 119, 178, 203–204, 210–211
  legitimization of, 177
Helplessness, 18, 35, 45, 115, 121, 154
High-risk areas, 11, 30–31, 33–34, 44, 45, 46, 47, 54, 194, 197
Holocaust, the, 138, 140–141, 191
Holocaust survivors, xvi, 18–19, 138–154
  and aging, 142, 150
  and anxiety, 144–149, 153–154
  blaming of, 151
  clinical population, 149, 174, 182–183
  and coping, 142
  and distress, 145–149
  and fear, 146
  and helplessness, 154
  nonclinical population, 149–151
  and panic, 146
  and perception of danger, 145
  and PTSD, 142
  reactivation, 138–139, 150, 152, 153, 182
  and self-efficacy, 145–149
  unresolved grief, 150
  vulnerability, 141, 142–143, 146, 149–151, 152
"Home front," the, 197
Hospital admission, 48–50
  psychiatric, 174–175, 181
  social services, 50–51

Impact of Event Scale (IES), 161–165, 167
Indirect tolerance, 143
Intifada, 29, 137
  and children, 117–118
Israel Defense Forces (IDF), 18, 26, 48, 66, 82, 88, 191–212, 217
  Civil Defense Force, 206–207
  Department of Behavioral Science (DBS), 36, 46, 48, 54, 60, 93, 94, 134
  faith in, 46, 48, 134, 195

Psychiatric patients (*cont.*)
  hospitalized, 177–178
  improvement, 184
  medication consumption, 184, 186–187, 188–189
  panic, 178, 186
  paranoia, 178, 179, 182
  psychoses, 174
  regression, 173
  restraint, 186–187
  schizophrenia, 183, 185, 186–186, 188, 190
  somatic complaints, 183
  vulnerability, 174, 189

Recovery environment, 171. *See also* Postwar environment
Research in wartime, viii, x, xv, xvi, 23–24, 36, 159, 189–190

Saddam Hussein, 1, 2, 3, 4, 5, 17, 18, 20, 86, 139, 177
"Saddam Syndrome," 178
Schools, 14, 15, 16, 82, 102–103, 216
Scuds. *See* Missile attacks
Sealed room, xvi, 5, 6, 7–8, 10, 11, 12, 13–14, 16, 31, 58, 63, 72, 121
  compliance, 45
  and the family, 63
  and Holocaust survivors, 139
  somatic reactions in, 43
  *See also* Protective devices; Shelter
Secondary gain, 160. *See also* War
Shelter, 13, 14, 16, 17, 18, 31. *See also* Protective devices; Sealed room
Singles, 77
Sirens, 8, 10, 11, 12, 13, 16
  warning time, 12, 16
Six Day War, xiii, xiv, xv, 4, 8, 30, 137, 140–141, 208, 220
Sleep disturbances, 30–32, 54, 179
  actigraph, 31
  and the elderly, 135
  "environmental insomnia," 31
  and gender, 92–93
  infants, 108
  soldiers, 202

Social causation hypothesis, 170
Social drift hypothesis, 170
Social functioning
  and the elderly, 135
Social support, 125, 127, 200–202, 205
Sociodemographic status, 163–171
Soldiers (Israeli), xvii, 191–212
  and anxiety, 197, 207
  and behavioral stress effects, 194
  and cognitive stress effects, 194, 202
  and coping, 195, 200–201, 205
  and denial, 208
  and depression, 207
  and distress, 199–202, 207
  and emotional stress effects, 194
  and functioning, 207–208
  and hypersensitivity, 200
  and hypervigilance, 200, 202
  and intrusion, 202
  and morale, 196
  and panic, 202
  and perceived danger, 200–201
  and PTSD symptoms, 199
  and rank, 198
  and reactivation, 208–210
  and regressive behavior, 207
  and self-efficacy, 200–202, 205
  and sense of safety, 196
  and sleep disturbances, 202
  and somatic stress effects, 194, 202
  and stress-related symptoms, 199–202
  and tension, 196
  use of time, 197
Solidarity, family, 60–61
Somatic complaints, 44, 47, 54, 94, 169, 183, 194, 202
Stress evaporation, 117, 125, 128
Stress inoculation perspective, 143, 217–218
Stress residuals, 117, 122, 125–126
Symptom Checklist (SCL-90), 161–165, 167, 199, 200, 202